THE CRUNCH FITNESS GUIDES

ON YOUR MARK. GET SET. GO! MARATHON TRAINING

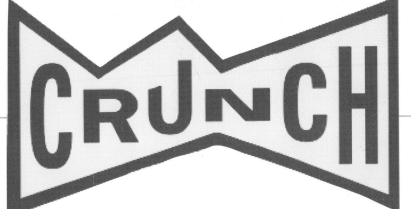

HATHERLEIGH

NEW YORK

Getfitnow.com Books
An Independent Imprint of Hatherleigh Press

Getfitnow.com Books
An Independent Imprint of Hatherleigh Press
an affiliate of W.W. Norton & Company
500 Fifth Avenue
New York, NY 10110
1-800-367-2550
www.getfitnow.com

Before beginning any strenuous exercise program consult your physician. The author and publisher of this book and workout disclaim any liability, personal or professional, resulting from the misapplication of any of the training procedures described in this publication.

All GetFitNow.com books are available for bulk purchase, special promotions, and premiums. For more information, please contact the manager of our Special Sales department at 1-800-367-2550.

Library of Congress Cataloging-in-Publication Data

On your mark, get set, go! : marathon training / Crunch.
        p.cm. -- (Crunch fitness guides)
      ISBN 1-57826-050-7
      1. Marathon running--Training. I. Title: Marathon training. II. Crunch. III.
  · Crunch fitness series
      GV1065.17.173 059 2000
      796.42′52--dc21
                                                                99-087621

Printed in Canada

Series Editor: Heather Ogilvie
Cover design: Lisa Fyfe
Text design and composition: John Reinhardt Book Design
Photographs: Chia Messina

Printed on acid-free paper

10 9 8 7 6 5 4 3 2 1

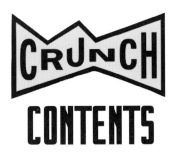

CONTENTS

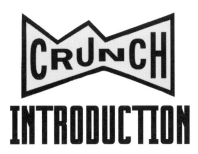

INTRODUCTION

Welcome to CRUNCH! For over a decade, we've been welcoming people of all shapes, sizes, ages, and fitness levels to our gyms. As we've expanded from a tiny, one-room aerobics studio in New York's East Village to cities across the country (and even to Tokyo), we've offered group fitness classes, personal training, and equipment to appeal to everyone from stressed-out workaholics and jet setters to senior citizens and expectant moms. We're living up to our motto, "No Judgements!"

We're aware that some people shy away from joining a gym or from starting a fitness program because they think it demands too great a change in their lifestyle. But at CRUNCH, we believe you shouldn't have to change your lifestyle in order to be fit. In fact, we believe your workout should change to fit your lifestyle. It is our firm belief that the success of a fitness program has nothing to do with how many hours you spend in the gym, but how good you feel when you're outside the gym, living your life.

That's why we've created these guides—to show you that no matter what your lifestyle, there's a workout you can do that will complement it and get you fit. For example, we designed the *Road Warrior Workout* for people who spend a lot of time traveling on business. These folks don't have to give up their fitness programs—in fact, by doing a workout specially adapted to life on the road, they can maintain their fitness level and become less susceptible to all the common aches and discomforts of travel.

Get Fit in a CRUNCH is for those people who are trying to shape up in time for a big event—a wedding, a reunion, a trip to the beach. Based on CRUNCH's popular class, Emergency Beach Training, *Get Fit in a CRUNCH* lays out a safe, effective four-week workout, 12-week workout, and six-month workout.

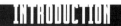

Since the hardest part of any fitness program is starting it, we've written *Beginner's Luck* to help people stay motivated and become more familiar with—and less intimidated by—basic cardiovascular and strength training exercises. It's a workout you can take at your own pace, according to your own goals.

Other CRUNCH guides include *The Workaholic's Workout*, targeting time-pressed workaholics; *On Your Mark. Get Set. Go! Marathon Training*, for first-time marathon runners; and *Posture Perfect*, for people who want to eliminate or avoid common back pain and improve posture.

At CRUNCH, we don't want you to conform to some workout fad or a lifestyle of spending more time at the gym than at play. We want to give you workout options that will conform to your lifestyle—without judgement.

Doug Levine
Founder and CEO
Crunch Fitness International, Inc.
www.crunch.com

CRUNCH
ABOUT THE AUTHOR

Kevin Oriol, personal trainer, group fitness instructor, and kickboxing instructor (A.C.E., I.S.S.A.) was, in his words, fat and out of shape some 7 years ago. A friend at work convinced him to run a 3.1-mile race during which he claims he felt as if he would die. After the ordeal he vowed to get in shape. A little over one year later, he completed his first marathon, losing 45 pounds along the way. Since then Kevin has completed 4 marathons, 9 half marathons, 8 triathlons, 3 biathlons, 1 bicycle century, and 25 other races varying in distances from 3.1 miles to 18 miles. Never coming in first, but never finishing last,

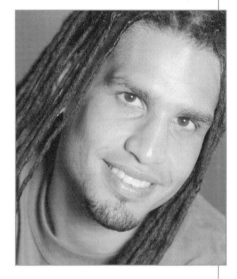

Kevin competes for the joy of the challenge and the many benefits of the exercise. His training tips have been published in the health section of *Elle Magazine*.

When Kevin is not training himself or his clients, you might find him at one of New York City's local rock clubs fronting his hard core band "Kill By Inches."

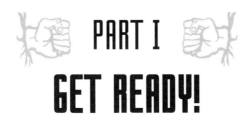

PART I
GET READY!

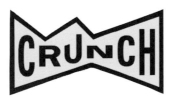

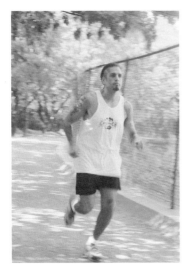

What's a good test of peak physical health? Some people might say a stress test at a doctor's office. Others might say winning a five-set tennis match, keeping up with a bunch of kids on a basketball court, or just plain feeling good and having the energy to do all the things you want to do every day.

Then there are runners. For a large percentage of this crowd, testing physical ability means bringing themselves to the brink of collapse—collapse from exhaustion, dehydration, energy depletion, muscle trauma, bone stress....The ultimate test for these folks is the marathon.

For such an extreme test of physical—and mental—prowess, the marathon seems a little arbitrary: Why 26.2 miles? For the answer, you have to go back over 2000 years to the plains of Marathon in Greece. Athenians had to defend the plains of Marathon from a surprise invasion from the Persians. Caught unawares and without any help, the Athenians defeated the invaders in an overwhelming victory. From the battle-

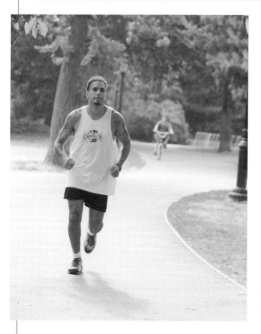

field, an Athenian general sent a messenger by foot to Athens, roughly 26.2 miles away, to deliver the news of victory. According to legend, the messenger made it to Athens, delivered his message of victory, then collapsed and died.

Marathoners have been honoring the messenger's journey ever since—by trying to survive it.

While running is an excellent cardiovascular exercise to achieve and maintain optimum health, running a marathon—especially if you haven't trained correctly—is, well, not exactly *healthy*. As legend teaches us, it can kill you. Running 26.2 miles in one day takes its toll on even the most fit of athletes. But it's a challenge. And finishing a marathon is a badge of honor in our society.

You may want to run your first marathon so you can wear that badge. Or maybe you want to push your body to its peak performance. Or maybe you love running and competition and foresee running, even winning, future marathons, after your first. No matter what your motivation, you need to prepare yourself physically and mentally for the run. In the days of Porches, Concordes, and bullet trains, 26.2 miles may not seem very far, but believe me, it's a very long journey when your feet meet the street.

Because marathons have become so popular, over the years lots of people have shared their experiences about running and training for a marathon. We're going to cover basics everyone follows (never do a 26.2-mile run before the race, load up on carbohydrates before running, cross-train, buy good shoes, etc.) and give you some expert training tips that will not only help you go the distance on race day, but keep you in good shape for your *next* physical challenge....

FIRST TIME IS A CHARM?

Eager and naïve, first-time marathoners tend to run a huge risk of overtraining. When your training schedule says to run 3 miles one day, don't be tempted to run 4 just because you feel you can. *Stick to the schedule!* Overtraining will only set you back in the long run.

You may have heard that some Olympic marathoners train by running over 100 miles a week. You are *not* an Olympian! These athletes have been training their whole lives, and they are training to win—you just want to finish! The most you will run in one week during our 6-month training period is 36 miles. If you try to do more, you will most likely injure yourself, and the marathon finishing line will be that much farther away.

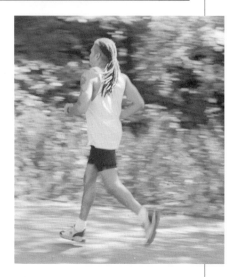

Before you start the actual training for your first marathon, you need to get the basics of marathon training down. To get the maximum benefit out of our 6-month training regimen, you also have to meet two minimum requirements:

1. Be able to jog 1 mile without stopping.
2. Have the desire and commitment to maintain your focus on your goal throughout your training.

As you might suspect, marathon training is not something you can do when you have a free hour here or there. It takes a great deal of time, so you need to make a regular time commitment. You might have to get up an hour earlier, even—or especially—on the weekends, which means you can't stay out late at night. You might have to forgo some parties and other late-night invitations. If you travel a lot, you might research your options for where you can run at your destination before you leave. In fact, your whole lifestyle can change to accommodate your training needs!

DEVELOP A FOOT FETISH

Your feet are going to take a pounding way before you run your first marathon. Be good to them. Shop at a reputable sports store and invest in a good pair of running shoes and a sports insert. There are different types of sneakers for your style of running (e.g., over-pronating, under-pronating, or normal) so don't purchase a sneaker just because it looks good. Also, most manufacturers use a cheap insert to keep the overall price of the sneaker low, so invest the extra $15 to $30 in a running insert. Your feet will be thanking you after 26.2 miles, believe me!

A knowledgeable salesperson can help you get the best fit. Some guidelines are that the shoe should be snug (but not uncomfortable) around the ankle, heel, and width of the foot. The toes, on the other hand (or should I say, "on the other foot"?) should have a half-inch space from the front of the sneaker. Your foot will slide forward a bit as you run, so if the sneaker is too tight on the toes, you might not have such a great run (to say the least).

ASSESS YOUR INJURIES

Now is the time to get the doc's permission if you have a chronic problem—sore lower back, knee, ankle, etc. Even a body part like your shoulders or neck can come into play in your training. See a qualified physician or an athletic chiropractor for a thorough evaluation and recommendation for rehabilitative exercises. You might feel as if you're starting from ground zero but you'll be laying down a strong foundation for a glorious finish 26 some-odd miles later.

STRETCH YOURSELF

This requirement is a "no brainer." Stretching is a crucial component of long-distance running. After a 5- to 10-minute warm-up, stretch. You should always warm up before you stretch—light cardiovascular exercise releases synovial fluid, a lubricant for your muscles and tendons and makes them less prone to injury. Stretching cold muscles can lead to pulled muscles and other injuries.

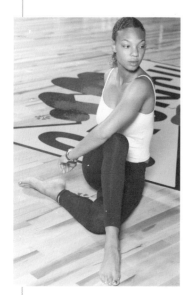

After you're done running or working out, stretch again. Once a week, take a yoga class. Not into yoga? Consider the following:

1. Where else are you going to get an intensive stretch for every part of your body for 60 to 75 minutes?

2. Yoga will teach you how to breathe properly and focus mentally. This will come in handy when you "hit the wall" at about mile 16, when the only thing that will keep you going is all the hard work you put in at training and your mental toughness. If you're serious about running a marathon, you'll take a yoga class . . . period.

BEGIN STRENGTH TRAINING

Our focus here will be on strengthening joints and ligaments and all major muscle groups. If you're inexperienced around the weight room, it might be a good time to invest in personal training. A good trainer will not only guide you through a routine that will help you improve your strength, but will teach you proper technique and form. Muscle groups to focus on include:

- Quadriceps/Glutes
- Hamstrings/Calves
- Abs/Lower Back
- Chest/Back
- Shoulders/Biceps/Triceps

Many people face a complete mystery when they consider using weights: How much should I lift and how many times? And once and for all, what the heck is a "rep"?

Well, let's try to clear up some of the confusion. "Rep" is short for repetition—how many times you consecutively execute the exercise. Sets are groups of reps. So if I say we will do 2 sets of 10 reps, that means we will lift the weight 10 times twice, with a brief (30-second) rest between sets.

How much weight should you use? Well, we lift weights to tire out the muscle. If you breeze through the exercises, and on a larger scale, the entire set, you won't get the most out of your weight training. When you do 15 reps, by the time you hit number 13 or 14, your muscles should be feeling it! Some weight-training exercises are body weight specific (for example, lifting half your weight on the leg press, which would be lifting 75 lbs. if you weigh 150 lbs.). (Keep in mind, though, that machines by different manufacturers will vary in weight resistance. I've found that 50 lbs. on one machine might feel lighter or heavier on another machine. Use common sense when weight training. Adjust the weight to be close to our rep goals.) For the most part, you'll use a weight that barely allows you to complete the set. If your life absolutely depended on it, you might be able to lift the weight 2 more times. Is that intense? Yes it is, as intense as 26.2 miles.

Rest time, between sets, will also be important in our training. Powerlifters will sometimes wait 3 to 5 minutes between sets to allow their bodies to "re-energize;" they are training for a short burst of absolute strength. Since we are training for endurance—the marathon—we'll train the body to sustain a relatively high heart rate for a long period of time; therefore, we'll rest between sets for only about 15 to 60 seconds.

FUEL FOR THE FLEET OF FOOT: WHAT TO EAT

As your training progresses, you'll need more and more calories to fuel your efforts. But just because you require more food doesn't mean you should eat whatever you want. The quality of the food is especially important to long-distance runners.

You want to provide your muscles with a steady supply of the most efficient energy source you can, and the most efficient fuel for running is carbohydrates. Now, you may be thinking, "Great—chocolate cake is a carbohydrate!" True, but it is a simple carbohydrate, and your muscles burn up simple carbs very quickly. Pasta, on the other hand, is a complex carbohydrate, which your muscles burn more slowly. Hence, marathoners tend to "carbo load" on pasta, pancakes, or bagels before they run.

A good runner's diet consists of 60% carbohydrate, 20% protein, and 20% fat. To approximate the total daily calories you need, multiply your body weight by 15. For example, a woman weighing 135 lbs. will start off ingesting 2025 calories. If in one week she gains any weight, she should lower her total calories by 300. She should continue this process until she maintains her weight.

The week before the marathon, you should be well hydrated—that means drinking plenty of water. You should also "carbo load" 2 to 3 days before the race (eat lots of pasta). Don't eat spicy food, high-fat foods (which take longer to digest), or food you've never had before. You do not want to disrupt your system with any surprises this week! On the day of the race, your breakfast should be very light. My favorite pre-marathon breakfast is toast and tea.

Hydration, of course, is of paramount importance. During the marathon, try to drink a little bit of water every mile for the first hour, then alternate between water and a sports drink (like Gatorade) for the rest of the race. Don't try to eat sports bars during the marathon unless you've done so without ill effects during your training.

After the marathon your body will be completely depleted of fuel and nutrients—eat whatever you want!

KEEP A TRAINING LOG

A training log is an invaluable tool. Recording your progress in a notebook that you can refer to will contribute to your sense of accomplishment. The log will become a source of motivation—challenging you to stick to your schedule and to figure out ways to overcome shortcomings in your training.

Here's how it works: At the beginning of each week record what you plan to do according to the program in this book (For ease, you can use the detailed training log provided in Appendix B). Then, every day, record what you actually did (e.g., how many miles you ran, what strength training exercises you did, or whether you took a yoga class). Record how you felt at the end of each run, where you ran, how long it took you, what the weather was like, and even what you ate. You'll be able to see where your training faltered—perhaps you need to eat more before a run; perhaps you need to drink more water or wear different clothes in certain weather conditions. You'll also see what workouts, running routes, foods, etc. are working for you.

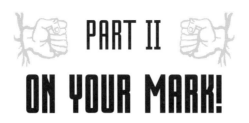

PART II
ON YOUR MARK!

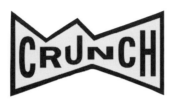

WEEKS 1-8

Your goal in the first few weeks is to build core strength and endurance and develop flexibility.

You will start training 5 days a week. During Weeks 1 through 4, you'll run 3 days, do weight training 1 day, and take a yoga class 1 day. For Weeks 5 to 8, you'll add another day of weight training.

The reps in our exercises are in the 15 to 20 range, meaning that the weights should be relatively light. Again, our goal is to start to strengthen all of the major muscle groups and the corresponding ligaments and tendons.

Before you do the strength training exercises you should do a 5- to 10-minute warm-up. You could jog, bike, jump rope, do jumping jacks, etc. You want to get your muscles a little warm. Then, just as on running days, you want to stretch. So before we describe each of the strength training exercises, let's review 12 basic stretches. Try to hold each stretch for 15 to 30 seconds.

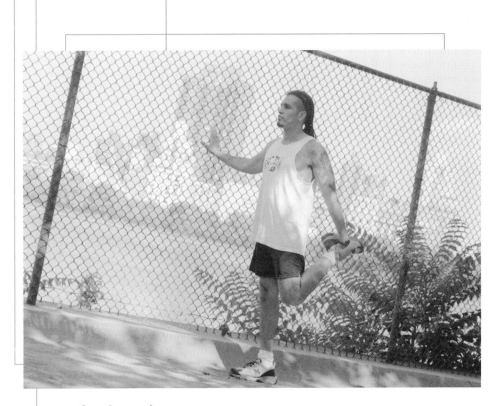

Quad stretch

With one hand, hold onto a stationary object for balance. Bend the opposite knee and with the free hand grab onto your ankle. Gently pull the ankle up toward your butt. Keep your thighs and knees parallel and your back straight. Do not swing your bent knee out to the side. Repeat with the opposite side.

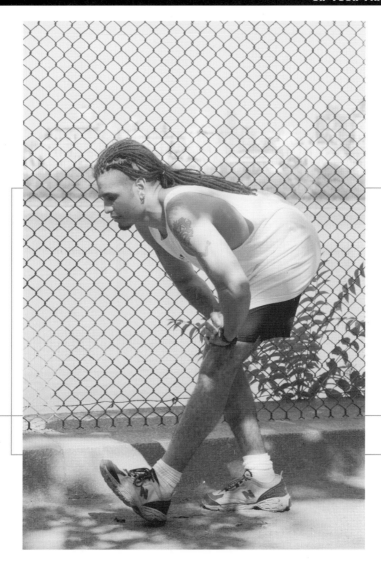

Hamstring stretch

Take a small step forward with one leg. Bend the opposite knee slightly and bend your torso down to a 45 degree angle to your hips. Repeat on the opposite side.

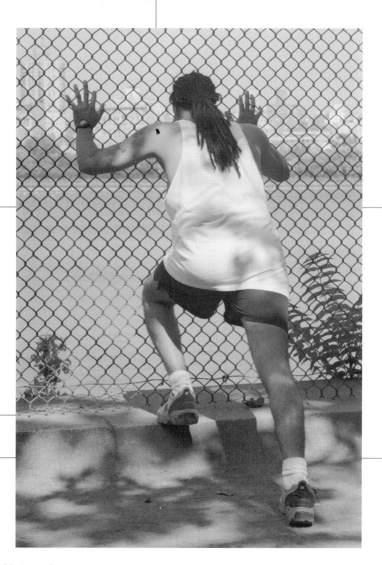

Calf stretch

Stand next to a wall, fence, or other stationary object. Take a large step back from the object, then fall forward toward it, keeping your heels on the ground. You can also lunge onto a step, as shown.

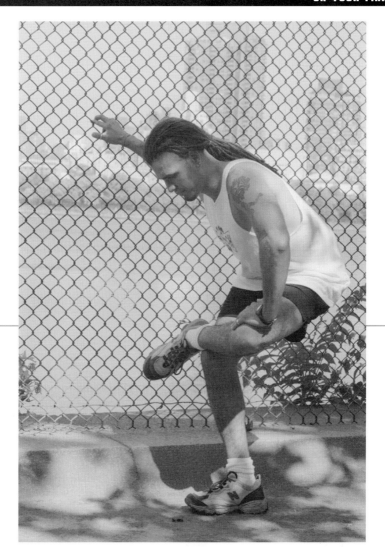

Glute stretch

While standing and holding a stationary object for balance, cross one ankle over the opposite knee, as shown. Lower your butt toward the ground, as if you were going to sit. Keep your back straight and your weight on your heel. Repeat with the opposite side.

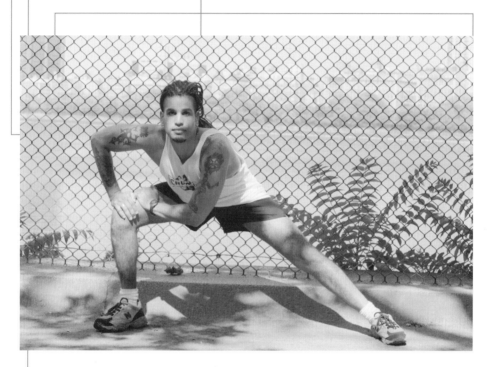

Inner thigh stretch

Stand straight and take a lunging step to the side with one leg. Bend into your knee while keeping your other leg firmly planted on the ground. Keep your butt back and the weight of your body on the bent leg's heel. Repeat on the opposite side.

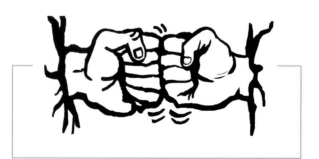

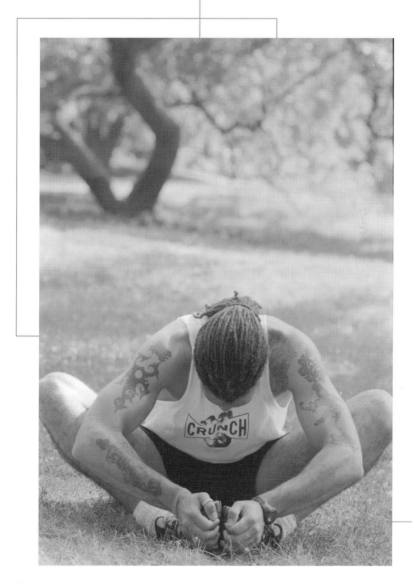

Butterfly stretch

Sitting on the ground with your feet touching and your knees out to the sides, lean your head, shoulders, and upper back forward.

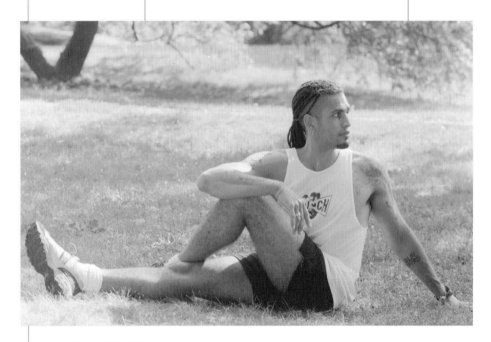

Spinal twist

Sit with your right leg straight out in front of you. Bend the left knee and place the left foot on the far side of the right knee. Turn your torso to the left. Repeat with the opposite side.

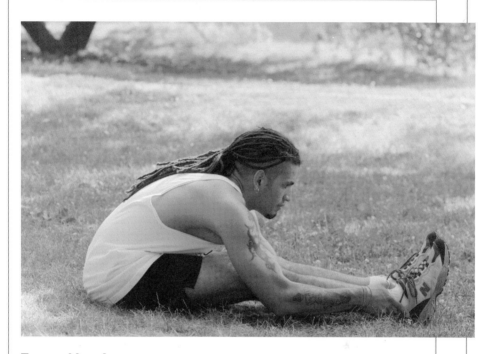

Forward bend

Sit with your legs straight out in front of you. Bend forward and reach for your ankles.

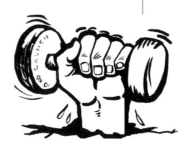

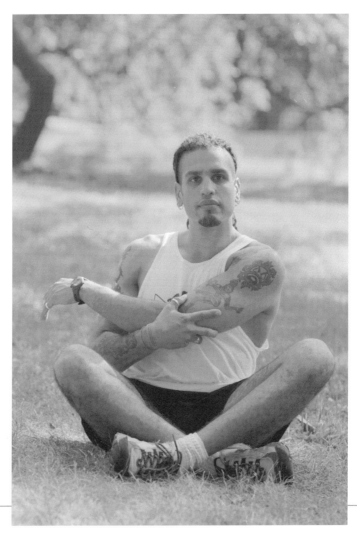

Shoulder stretch

Place your left arm on a diagonal across your chest. With your right arm, gently pull your left arm closer into your body. Repeat on the opposite side.

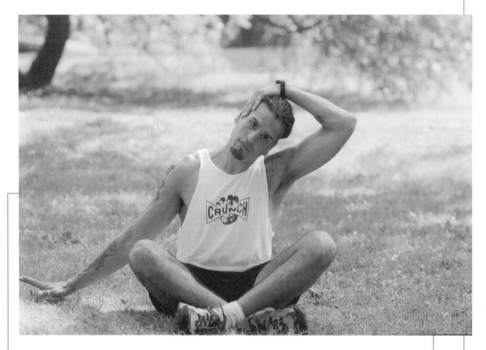

Neck stretch

Extend one arm out to the side. Feel as if you're pushing through the wrist. Place the other hand on the opposite side of your head and gently tilt your head. Do not bend your head back—doing so can damage the cartilage in your neck.

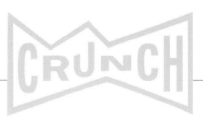

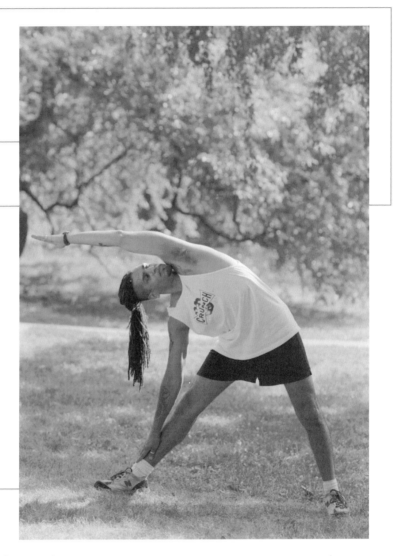

Side stretch

Stand with your legs wider than shoulder-width apart and bend your torso to your left side. With your right hand, grasp your right ankle, while stretching your left arm over your head to the left side. Repeat on the opposite side.

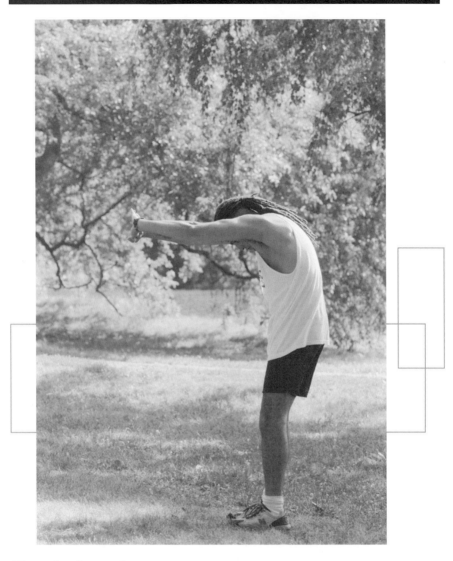

Upper back stretch

Stand with your arms out in front of you. Grasp your hands together, with palms facing outward. Crunch your abdominals, relax your head forward and reach forward through your wrists.

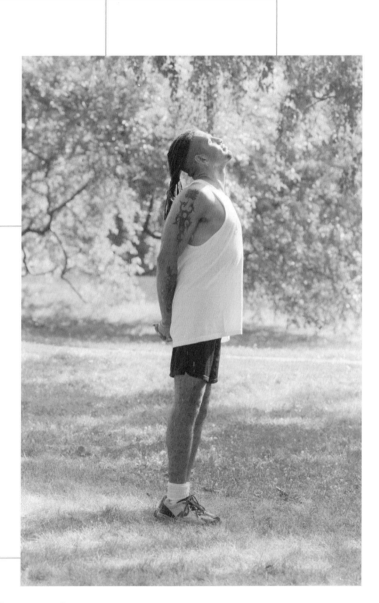

Chest stretch

Clasp hands together behind your back, relax your shoulders, and expand your ribcage upward.

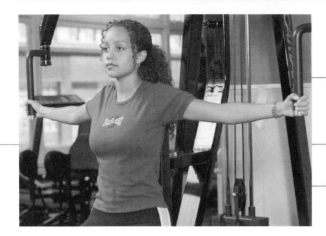

Now that you're stretched out, we'll describe the strength training exercises you'll be doing in these first few weeks. As you perform each exercise, keep in mind that you want to exhale on the "push," or hard part of the motion, and inhale on the easy part. For example, in a crunch, you want to exhale as you crunch up, and inhale as you go back down.

Also, bear in mind that machines vary from gym to gym, so always read the instructions on each machine before doing the exercise—as well as reading our tips for safe and effective exercises here.

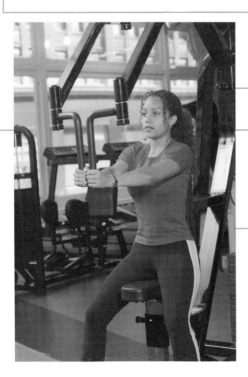

WEIGHT TRAINING ROUTINE FOR WEEKS 1–4

Muscles	Exercise	Sets/Reps*
Legs	Reverse lunges	2x20(each leg)
	Step-ups	2x20(each leg)
	Leg presses	2x10(1/2 your weight)
	Hamstring curls	2x15
Upper body	Push-ups	1 set until exhaustion
	Pec decks	2x20
	Weight-assisted pull-ups	1 set until exhaustion (½ your weight)
	Seated rows	2x20
	Shoulder presses	2x20
	Lateral raises	2x15
Abdominal	Crunches	200 (sets of 25 to 50 reps totaling 200)

*"2x20" means 2 sets of 20 reps.

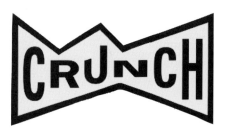

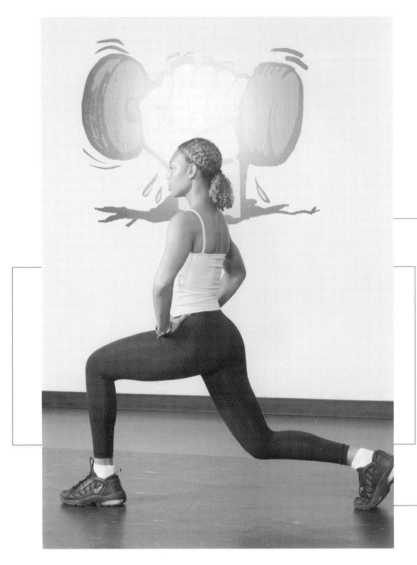

Reverse lunges

Stand straight with your hands on your hips. With your right leg, take a large step backward. Keep a 90° angle in the left leg and lift your body weight through your left heel. Alternate legs.

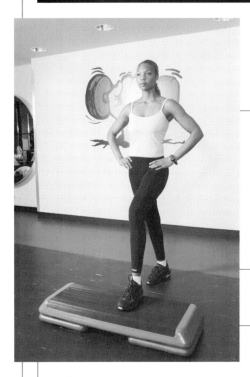

Step-ups

You can use steps or stairs or a flat bench surface. The step should be no higher than your hips. One foot should be el-evated on the step, while the second foot stays flat on the floor. The top leg extends from a near right angle (shin and thigh) to an almost straight leg. Don't lock your knee! Repeat with the opposite foot on the step.

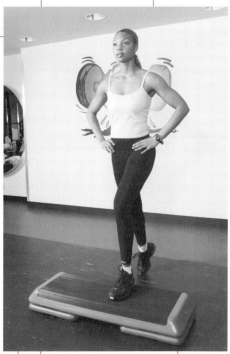

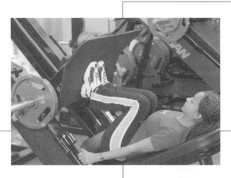

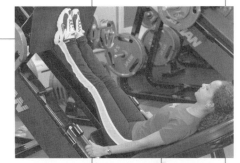

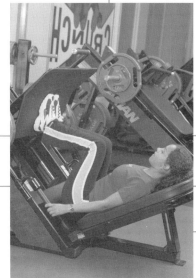

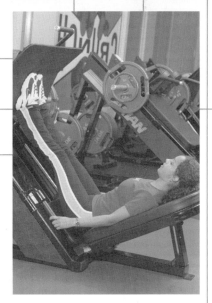

Leg presses

Sitting on the leg press, grab the handles at your sides. To start, place your feet wider than hip-width apart (to focus on inner thighs), at hip-width apart (to focus on overall thighs), or closer than hip-width apart (as shown, to focus on outer thighs). Be sure you feel your head, lower back, and hips on the seat. On an inhale, lower the weight slowly until your legs form a 90 degree angle, then exhale as you push through full feet to the starting position.

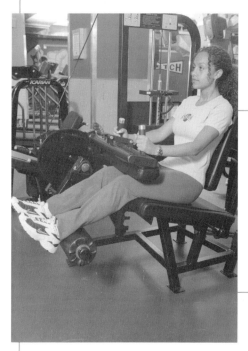

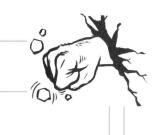

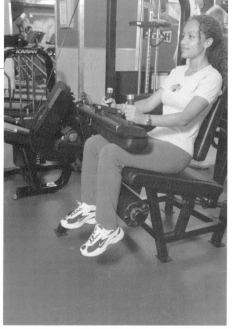

Hamstring curls

Sit on the leg curl machine and hold the hand grips. The pad should rest on the back of your ankles. Align the axis pin to the rear of your knee by adjusting your seat back accordingly. *This is very important!* If the axis pin is not aligned correctly, you could hurt your knees. Point your toes toward the ceiling and keep your back slightly flexed. Relax your feet and press the pad down so that a 90 degree angle is formed between your upper and lower legs.

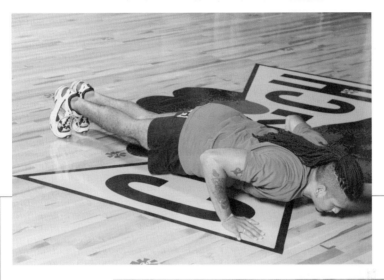

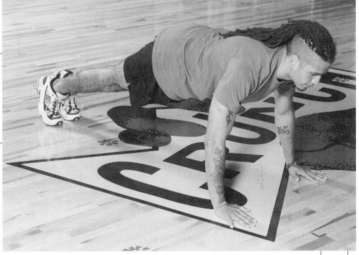

Push-ups

You can do these from your knees (with your feet in the air) or from your toes. In either case, place your hands slightly wider than shoulder-width apart. Keep your abs tight, your back flat (not swayed), and your head up. While push-ups mainly work the chest muscles, they also work the shoulders, triceps, and abs.

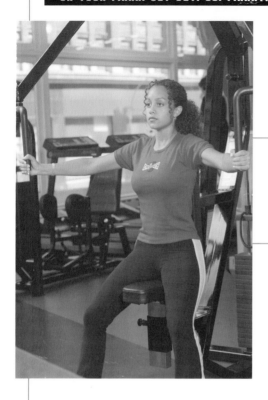

Pec decks

Sit on the bench between the handles, keep your back straight, and grab the handles. Your elbows should be bent back at a 45 degree angle and raised high, but lower than your shoulders. (Letting your elbows drop is bad for your shoulders.) Bring the handles together in front of you.

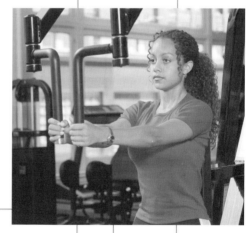

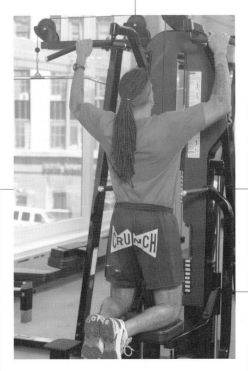

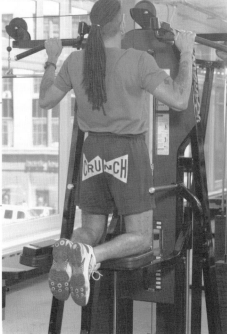

Weight-assisted pull-ups

The weight in this machine is designed to counterbalance your body
weight. Start off with a heavy weight
(half your body weight) and gradually decrease the weight until you're
able to do pull-ups without using a counterbalance. Note that some
machines, like the one pictured here, require you to kneel on the platform. There are others, however, that require you to stand on the platform. Either machine is effective. *Important:* Don't let go of the handles
until your knees (or feet) are off the platform, or else the platform will
crash to the bottom!

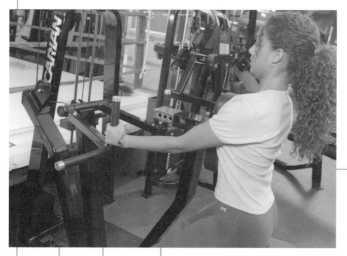

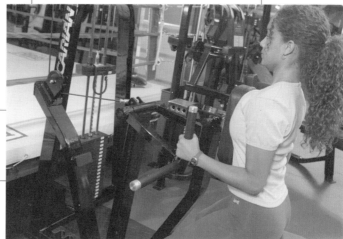

Seated rows

Keep your back straight and support yourself, rather than resting your chest on the chest pad. Don't round your shoulders forward. Grabbing the handles low, drive your elbows back, rather than pulling back with your hands.

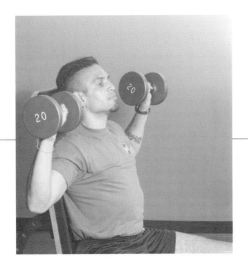

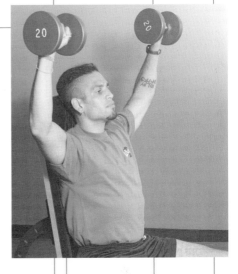

Shoulder presses

Sit on the bench with your feet flat on the floor and a dumbbell in each hand. Start with the dumbbells just above and outside of your shoulders. On an exhale, push the weight up and return to starting position with an inhale.

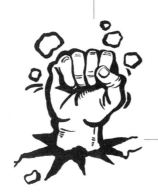

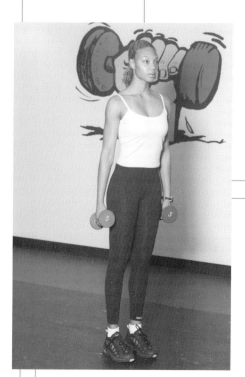
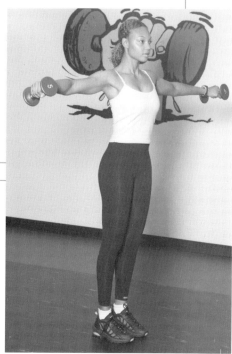

Lateral raises

Stand straight with your feet shoulder-width apart and knees slightly bent. Hold the dumbbells in your hands with your palms facing down, elbows slightly bent. Raise your arms slowly up to shoulder height, exhaling as you do so. Hold for two counts and slowly return to starting position, inhaling slowly. Do not raise the dumbbells over your shoulders, which will place stress on the shoulders and may injure the rotator cuff. Concentrate on moving your arms out laterally before lifting them straight up.

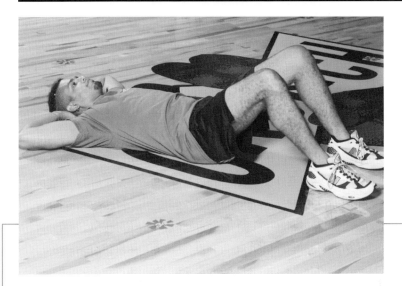

Crunches

Lie on your back on the floor with your knees bent up and your feet flat on the floor. Place your hands behind your head, but be careful not to pull your head and neck up—your head should just be resting in your hands. Crunch up, bringing your head toward your knees and slowly lowering it again—but not all the way to the floor! Keep your shoulder blades just off the floor. Do not crane up—think of raising your rib cage.

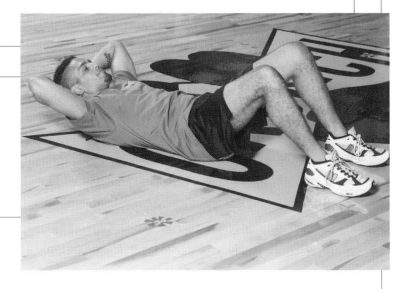

WEEK 1

Total mileage—5 miles

Mon:	Off
Tues/Thurs:	Run* 1 mile
Wed:	Weights
Fri:	Yoga
Sat or Sun:	Long run—3 miles**

*The word "run" is used, but jogging is fine. If you have a heart rate monitor (very useful), subtract your age from 190. You should not go above this number during your short runs (approximately 90% of your maximum heart rate, or MHR). Then subtract your age from 175. You should not go above this number during your long runs (approximately 80% of your MRH).

**This is you base. If you can't complete 3 miles without stopping, then run/walk until you can complete 3 miles without stopping.

WEEK 2

Repeat Week 1.

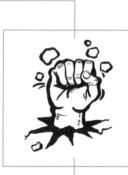

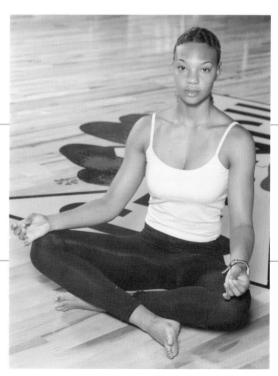

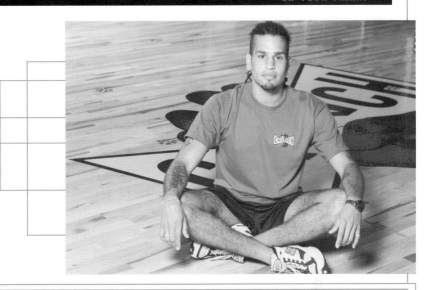

WEEK 3

Total mileage—6 miles

Mon:	Off
Tues:	Run 1 mile
Wed:	Weights
Thurs:	Run 2 miles
Fri:	Yoga
Sat or Sun:	Long run—3 miles

WEEK 4

Total mileage—8 miles

Mon:	Off
Tues:	Run 2 miles
Wed:	Weights
Thurs:	Run 2 miles
Fri:	Yoga
Sat or Sun:	Long run—4 miles

WEEK 5

Repeat Week 4 but make Saturday a weight day
and Sunday a long run.

WEIGHT TRAINING ROUTINE WEEKS 5—8 (2-DAY SPLIT)

WEDNESDAY

Muscles	Exercise	Sets/Reps
Legs	Reverse lunges	2 x 30 (alternating legs)
	Step-ups	2 x 30 (alternating legs)
	Leg presses	3 x 12 (½ your weight)
	Hamstring curls	3 x 15
Upper body	Shoulder presses	3 x 20
	Lateral raises	3 x 15
Abdominal	Crunches	200

SATURDAY

Muscles	Exercise	Sets/Reps
Legs	Calf raises	2 x 20
	Hip abductors	2 x 20
	Hip adductors	2 x 20
Upper body	Push-ups	2 sets until exhaustion
	Dumbbell bench presses	2 x 20
	Pec decks	2 x 20
	Weight-assisted pull-ups	2 sets until exhaustion (½ your weight)
	Seated rows	2 x 20
Abdominal	Crunches	200

For Weeks 5 to 8 we'll increase sets but keep the weight mostly the same. Since the volume of exercise has increased, we'll split our weight training into two days—hence the two-day split (now you can start to talk "gym slang" to all the muscle heads at the squat racks).

Following are descriptions of the new exercises you'll be doing.

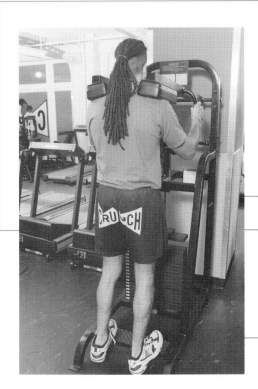

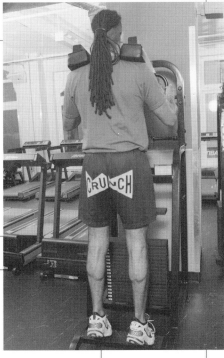

Calf raises

Adjust the shoulder pads on the machine so that they are at shoulder height when you're standing on the floor. Step up on the platform, grab the handles, and slide your shoulders under the pads. The balls of your feet should be on the platform, and your heels should clear the platform. Raise your heels up without bending your knees. Slowly lower your heels beneath platform level and repeat.

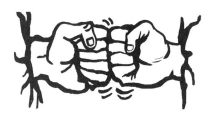

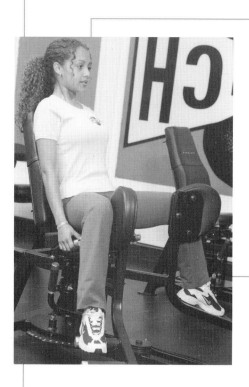

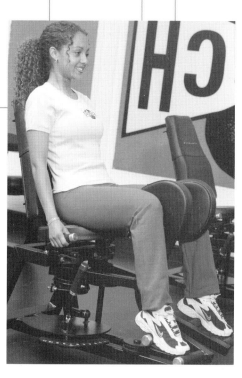

Hip abductors

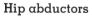

Sit on the machine so that your back is flat against the seat, grab the handles, and place your feet on the foot pegs so that your knees are bent at a 90 degree angle. Keep your abs strong. Squeeze the pads toward each other until your knees are close together. Slowly allow the pads to move outward, and return to the start position in a controlled movement.

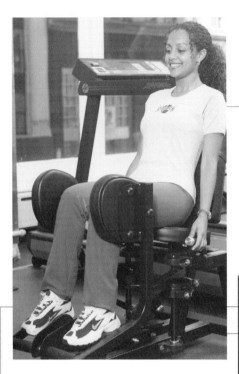

Hip adductors

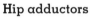

Sit on the machine so that your back is flat against the seat, grab the handles, and place your feet on the foot pegs so that your knees are bent at a 90 degree angle. Keep your abs strong. Slowly push the pads outward, moving the knees away from each other. Return to the start position in a controlled movement.

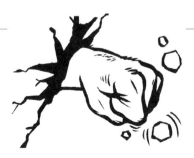

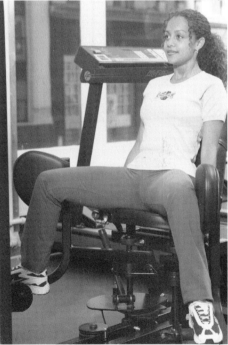

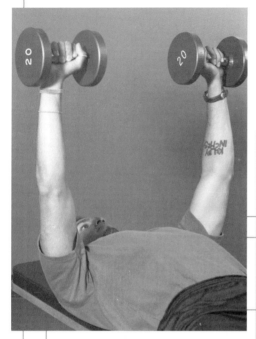

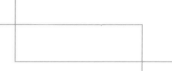

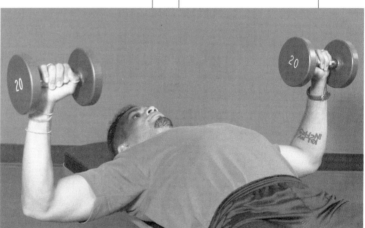

Dumbbell bench presses

Lie on your back on the bench and keep your feet either up on the bench or flat on the floor. Grasp dumbbells in each hand with palms facing away from you. To start, hold the dumbbells in fully extended arms over the mid-line of your chest. Bring the dumbbells down, bending your elbows. Do not drop your elbows below your body at the bottom, and do not lock your elbows at the top.

WEEK 6

Total mileage—9 miles

Mon:	Off
Tues:	Run 2 miles
Wed:	Weights
Thurs:	Run 3 miles
Fri:	Yoga
Sat:	Weights
Sun:	Long run—4 miles

WEEK 7

Total mileage—10 miles

Mon:	Off
Tues:	Run 3 miles
Wed:	Weights
Thurs:	Run 3 mile
Fri:	Yoga
Sat:	Weights
Sun:	Long run—4 miles

WEEK 8

Total mileage—11 miles

Mon:	Off
Tues:	Run 3 miles
Wed:	Weights
Thurs:	Run 3 miles
Fri:	Yoga
Sat:	Weights
Sun:	Long run—5 miles

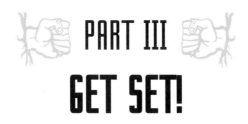

PART III
GET SET!

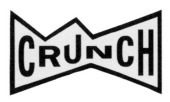

WEEKS 9 TO 16

Your goal in these weeks is to increase your cardiovascular endurance through cross training.

You will train 6 days a week during Weeks 9 to 12, tapering down to 5 days in Weeks 13 to 16 while increasing mileage slightly.

In this phase you'll be decreasing your running days and adding interval and cross training for 4 weeks. Decreasing running may seem strange, being that you want to increase mileage to at least 20 miles 1 to 3 times before the actual marathon. But since you'll be pounding the pavement in the last phase of your training, why not take this opportunity to continue to strengthen ligaments and muscle tissue while building up a stronger cardiovascular base for the long hours on the road? This is when you will finally get "in shape." You'll substitute days of running with other cardiovascular exercises/equipment to raise your anaerobic threshold. All runs should be at no more than 80 percent of your maximum heart rate (175 minus your age).

During cross training, your heart rate should be between 80 and 90 percent of your maximum heart rate. You may use any or all of the following activities to cross train:

Cycling:	45 minutes
	(outdoors or indoors*)
Swimming:	20–45 minutes
Rowing:	20–45 minutes
Stair Master:	20–45 minutes
Nordic Track:	20–45 minutes
Jumping Rope:	15–30 minutes

*Here's another "no brainer:" take a spin class! You'll get 45 minutes of great music and challenging intervals—perfect for these 4 weeks of higher intensity workouts. If the thought of being on yet another machine other than a treadmill mortifies you, then take any moderate- to high-intensity group class (e.g., step, sculpt, kickboxing, hip hop/dance, or anything that gets your heart range between 80 and 90 percent). Have fun, but remember that you still must work hard.

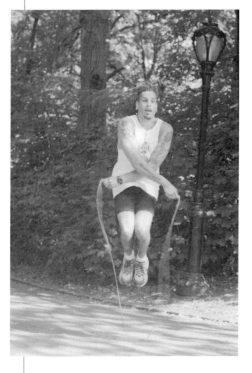

The interval training in this "Get Set" portion is an extension of the weight training of the first 8 weeks. Here we'll add calisthenics into the mix. You'll do exercises like jumping jacks, squat thrusts, push-ups, and vertical hops (all of the exercises that your high school coach tortured you with) in 1- to 3-minute intervals. This is intense training that will raise your anaerobic threshold, allowing you to feel stronger (greater cardiac output with less effort) in the last phase of your training.

A personal trainer might be key here, ensuring that (a) you do the exercises correctly, and (b) that you do the exercises. By your twelfth week of training, you should feel confident and strong in running 6 miles and the yoga should have increased your flexibility and balance. This is the foundation that will take you across the finish line on race day.

INTERVAL TRAINING FOR WEEKS 9 TO 12 (TWO-DAY SPLIT)

TUESDAY

Exercise	Sets/Reps/Time
Walking lunges	3 minutes
Leg presses	1 x 15 (½ your weight—e.g., if you weigh 120, lift 60 lbs. or adjust the weight to complete 15 reps.)
Leg presses	2 x 8 (your full body weight)
Jumping jacks	1 minute
Leg extensions	2 x 15
Vertical (or lateral) hops	1 minute
Push-ups	1 set until exhaustion
Incline bench presses	2 x 12
Push-ups	1 set until exhaustion
Bicep curls	2 x 15
Crunches	300

FRIDAY

Exercise	Sets/Reps/Time
Weight-assisted pull-ups	1 set until exhaustion (½ your weight)
Squat thrusts	1 minutes
Weight-assisted pull-ups	1 set until exhaustion (½ your weight)
Step-ups	2 minutes
Seated rows	2 x 15
Hamstring curls	1 x 15
Plié squats	1 x 25 (using a 10 to 25 lb. free weight)
Hamstring curls	1 x 15
Plié squats	1 x 25 (using a 10 to 25 lb. free weight)
Shoulder presses	2 x 15
Lateral raises	2 x 15
Calf raises	2 x 15
Crunches	300

The following are descriptions of the new exercises you'll be doing.

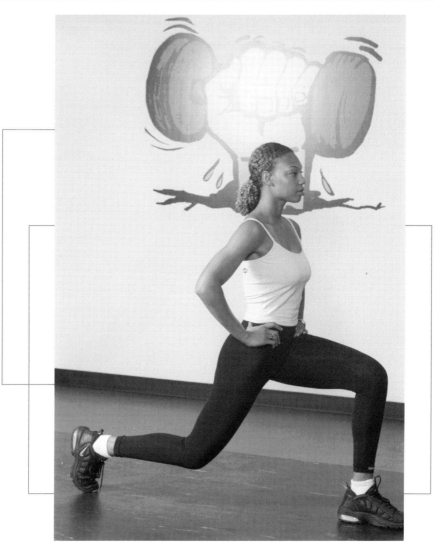

Walking lunges

Standing straight up with hands on hips, lunge to full stride with left foot and lower right knee close to the ground. Stand up again, moving forward, and lunge with your right foot. Travel forward in this manner for 3 minutes. (Pay no attention to the weird looks you'll get as you walk up and down the gym floor. If anyone asks what you are doing, yell "MARATHON TRAINING, BABY!")

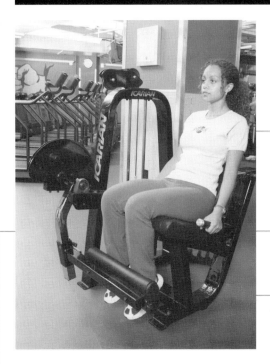

Leg extensions

Sit on the leg extension machine and grab the bars with both hands. Make sure the axis pin on the machine is aligned with the rear of your knee joint by adjusting the seat back accordingly. This is very important to avoid injury to your knee! The shin pad should rest just above the front ankles. Extend your legs fully, but do not lock your knee at the top. Do not bring the weight all the way down between reps.

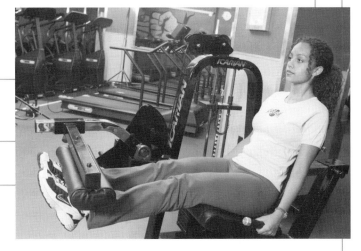

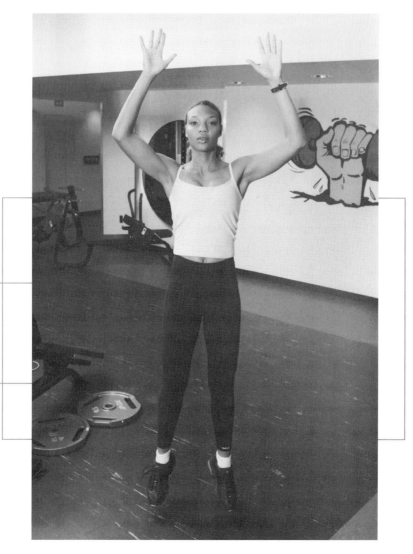

Vertical hops

Stand straight with a slight bend in your knees. Your arms should be bent at the elbow, fingers pointing up, palms facing forward. Jump up, extending your hands toward the ceiling.

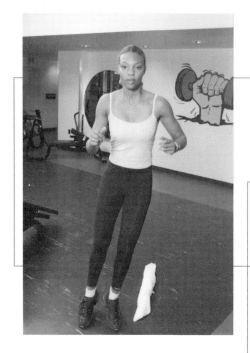

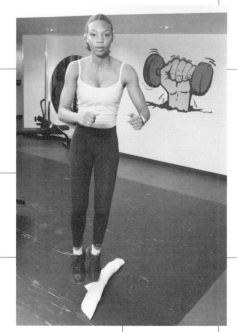

Lateral hops

Place a towel or jumprope on the ground beside you. Stand with your hands on your hips and a slight bend in your knees. Hop over the towel (or jumprope), back and forth. Keep your knees bent—think of a skier's position skiing over moguls.

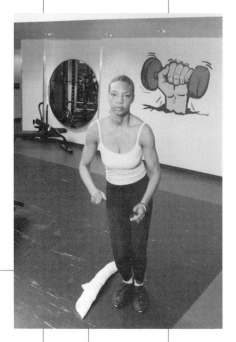

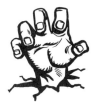

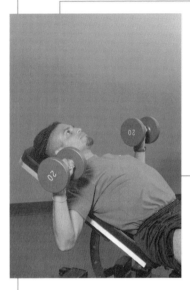

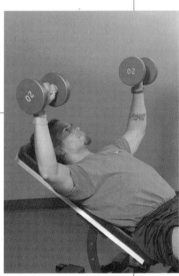

Incline bench presses

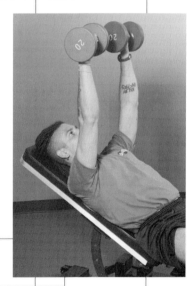

Lie on your back on a bench inclined to a 45 degree angle. Keep your feet flat on the floor. Grasping dumbbells in each hand with palms facing away from you, bend elbows so that they rest just below your back level. Raise dumbbells straight up until your arms are fully extended above you. Bring the dumbbells down again to just above your chest.

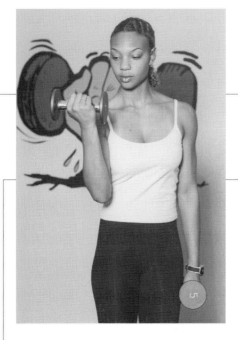

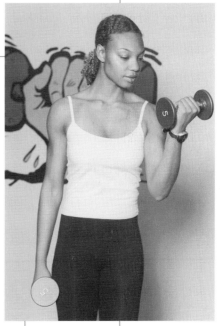

Bicep curls

Put your elbows at your sides and face your palms up. Lower the dumbbell toward the floor and then curl the dumbbell up to your shoulders.

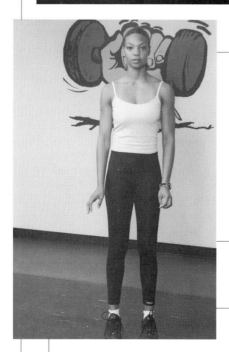

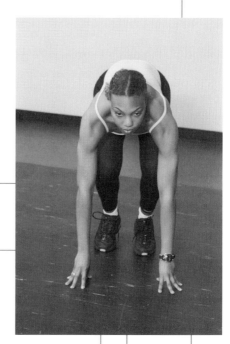

Squat thrusts

Stand straight with your arms at your sides. Bend your knees and place your hands on the floor in front of you. With your weight resting on your hands, kick your legs back to a fully extended position, then bring them back beneath your butt, and stand up again, using your legs, not your lower back. This is one squat thrust.

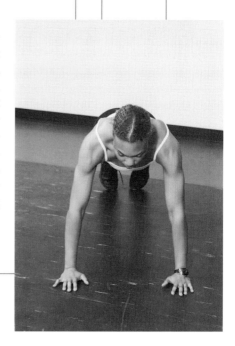

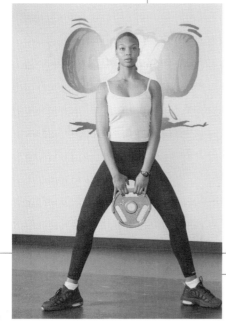 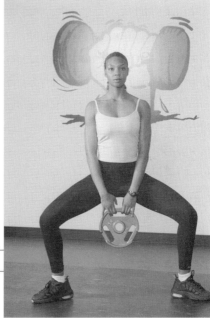

Plié squats

With your toes pointing outward and heels just outside shoulder-width apart, hold a weight in front of your body. Keep your glutes tight and lower your butt until your lower legs and thighs are at right angles. Raise back up and avoid locking your knees.

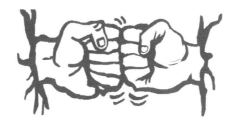

WEEK 9

Total mileage—8 miles

Mon:	Off
Tues:	Interval Training
Wed:	Run 3 miles
Thurs:	Cross Training
Fri:	Interval Training
Sat:	Yoga
Sun:	Run 5 miles

WEEK 10

Total mileage—9 miles

Mon:	Off
Tues:	Interval Training
Wednesday:	Run 4 miles
Thursday:	Cross Training
Friday:	Interval Training
Saturday:	Yoga
Sun:	Run 5 miles

WEEK 11

Total mileage—10 miles

Mon:	Off
Tues:	Interval Training
Wed:	Run 5 miles
Thurs:	Cross Training
Fri:	Interval Training
Sat:	Yoga
Sun:	Run 5 miles

WEEK 12

Total mileage—12 miles

Mon:	Off
Tues:	Interval Training
Wed:	Run 6 miles
Thurs:	Cross Training
Fri:	Interval Training
Sat:	Yoga
Sun:	Run 6 miles

INTERVAL TRAINING FOR WEEKS 13 TO 16

WEDNESDAY

Exercise	Sets/Reps/Time
Walking lunges	3 minutes
Leg presses	3x12 (your full body weight)
Squat thrusts	1 minute
Weight-assisted pull-ups	1 set until exhaustion (½ your weight)
Bicep curls	2x12
Vertical hops	1 minute
Push-ups	1 set until exhaustion
Flat bench presses	2x10
Mountain climbers	1 minute
Hamstring curls	2x12
Plie squats	2x25 (using a 10 –25 lb. free weight)
Jumping jacks	2 minutes
Crunches	300

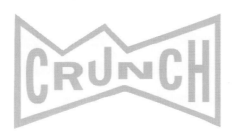

Here's a description of the new exercise you'll be doing.

MOUNTAIN CLIMBERS

Begin on the floor in the top of the push-up position and bring one knee up to your chest. Keeping a constant motion, alternate pumping your knees into your chest (like a runner's motion). Pay particular attention to keeping your back straight and arms soft enough to absorb shock.

This is the peak of your intensity training. This workout is hard on the muscular and cardiovascular systems. Since there are many jumping exercises, you should pay special attention to your footwear (cross-training sneakers are much better than running sneakers here), form, and enough space to execute these exercises safely. You should go through these exercises with as little rest as possible in between sets. A great way to measure progress is to record how much time it takes you to complete all of the exercises. The better your time, the more fit you are.

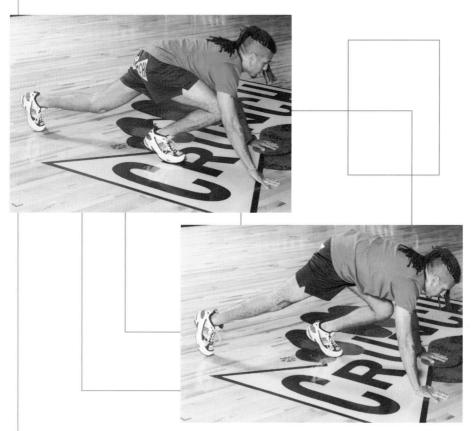

WEEK 13

Total mileage—12 miles

Mon:	Off
Tues:	Interval Training
Wed:	Run 5 miles
Thurs:	Off
Fri:	Cross Training
Sat:	Yoga
Sun:	Run 7 miles

WEEK 14

Total mileage—13 miles

Mon:	Off
Tues:	Interval Training
Wed:	Run 5 miles
Thurs:	Off
Fri:	Cross Training
Sat:	Yoga
Sun:	Run 8 miles

WEEK 15

Total mileage—14 miles

Mon:	Off
Tues:	Interval Training
Wed:	Run 6 miles
Thurs:	Off
Fri:	Cross Training
Sat:	Yoga
Sun:	Run 8 miles

WEEK 16

Total mileage—15 miles

Mon:	Off
Tues:	Interval Training
Wed:	Run 6 miles
Thurs:	Off
Fri:	Cross Training
Sat:	Yoga
Sun:	Run 9 miles

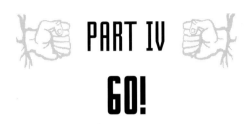

PART IV
GO!

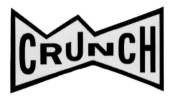

WEEKS 17 TO 24

Your goal in this phase of training is to improve your running endurance and maintain strength and flexibility.

You'll be training 6 days a week for Weeks 17 to 23, with the exception of Week 20. You'll be weight training until Week 22 and introducing massage as a part of your recovery days. You'll start to taper your running in the last two weeks. Tapering is a time-tested method of reserving your best effort for the race.

Around Week 18 or 19, when your long run is over 10 miles, you might consider running a 5K–10K race as part of your long run. This will help get the jitters out and mentally prepare you for the big race. After the 5K or 10K, take a few minutes to stretch. Then finish your long run at a slow and relaxed pace.

A WORD ABOUT MASSAGE

Massage helps to stimulate blood flow to muscles, loosen tight muscles, relieve tension, and promote relaxation. It also helps to eliminate lactic acid, a chemical waste product that builds up in muscle tissue during exercise.

Swedish massage is the most popular form of massage therapy. The therapist manipulates muscles lightly or deeply, depending on your comfort level.

While Swedish massage focuses on muscle manipulation, Shiatsu massage is energy oriented. The therapist locates and stimulates specific energy pressure points on the body. This increase of energy flow in the body assists the functioning of internal organs.

Reflexology focuses on loosening joints in the hands and feet to clear blockages along the energy meridiens that lead to the body's vital organs.

WEIGHT TRAINING FOR WEEKS 17 TO 22

Exercise	Sets/Reps
Bench presses	2 x 20
Lat pull-downs	2 x 20
Leg presses	2 x 15
Hamstring curls	2 x 15
Shoulder presses	2 x 15
Calf raises	2 x 15
Bicep curls	2 x 20
Tricep bench dips	2 sets to exhaustion

The following are descriptions of the new exercises you'll be doing.

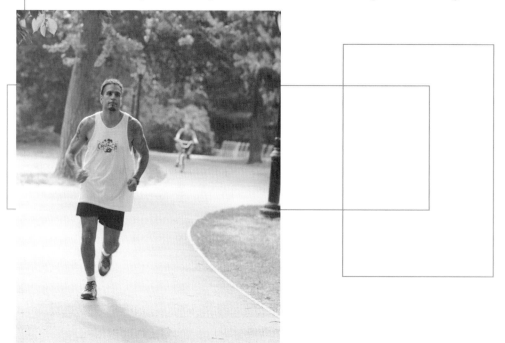

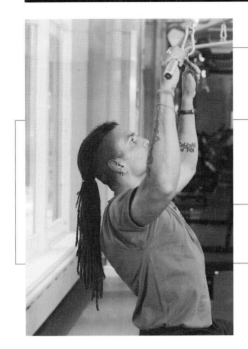
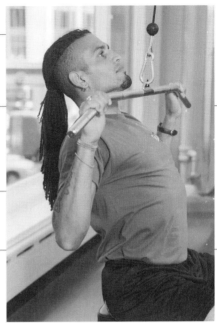

Lat pull-downs

Sit with the pad above your thighs. With a shoulder-width overgrip, pull the bar to the top of your collar bone while focusing on bringing your elbows straight down. Keep your back straight. Do *not* pull down or press down behind your head—you can injure your shoulder. Unfortunately, this is a very common mistake among gym members.

RACING TIPS

- Hold yourself back in the beginning. Don't be tempted to keep pace with other runners who are probably running too fast at the start. You want to conserve your energy for later in the race.

- Do not try to "push through" the "wall"—slow down and hydrate. Most runners hit the wall around mile 16.

- Run in a straight line, especially at the start. Weaving in and out of other runners can cause accidents.

- While running, you may get a cramp in your side, or what runners call a "stitch." It's caused by irregular breathing and affects your diaphragm muscle. You'll feel an annoying little pain between your ribcage and upper abdominal area. Slow down and try to breathe deeper. If it persists, walk and massage the cramped area. Breathe deeply to restore oxygen to the muscle and hydrate with water or a sports drink.

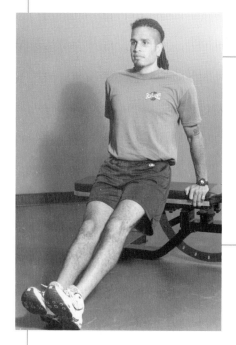

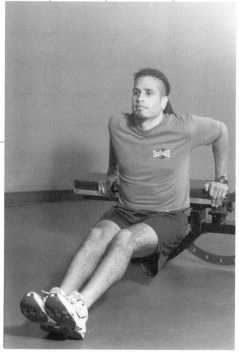

Tricep bench dips

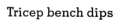

Sit on the edge of a bench and grasp the edge of the bench on either side of your hips with your hands. Raise your butt up and slightly forward off the bench. Keep your knees straight and keep your weight on your heels, while lowering your butt toward the floor. Raise back up. Keep your back flat and close to the edge of the bench. For an easier dip, you can bend your knees.

SIGNS OF DEHYDRATION

If you experience any of the following symptoms during a long run or during a marathon, stop! You are dehydrated and need water, shade, and medical attention.

- Dizziness
- Nausea
- Severe cramping
- Disorientation

- Headache
- Blurred vision
- Fainting

Since you're trying only to maintain muscle strength in this final phase, weights will decrease, similar to your first phase. We still want to work hard, but the focus should be on your running. You'll work through your sets and then stretch out in yoga class—mentally preparing for Saturday's long run.

WEEK 17

Total mileage—25 miles

Mon:	Massage
Tues:	Run 4 miles
Wed:	Run 4 miles
Thurs:	Run 4 miles
Fri:	Weight Training and Yoga
Sat:	Run 10 miles
Sun:	Run 3 miles

WEEK 18

Total Mileage—35 miles

Mon:	Off
Tues:	Run 6 miles
Wed:	Run 6 miles
Thurs:	Run 6 miles
Fri:	Weight Training and Yoga
Sat:	Run 14 miles
Sun:	Run 3 miles

WEEK 19

Total mileage—36 miles

Mon:	Massage
Tues:	Run 6 miles
Wed:	Run 4 miles
Thurs:	Run 6 miles
Fri:	Weight Training and Yoga
Sat:	Run 16 miles
Sun:	Run 4 miles

WEEK 20

Total mileage—32 miles

Mon:	Off
Tues:	Run 4 miles
Wed:	Run 4 miles
Thurs:	Run 4 miles
Fri:	Weight Training and Yoga
Sat:	Run 20 miles
Sun:	Off

WEEK 21

Total mileage—33 miles

Mon:	Massage
Tues:	Run 4 miles
Wed:	Run 6 miles
Thurs:	Run 4 miles
Fri:	Weight Training and Yoga
Sat:	Run 16 miles
Sun:	Run 3 miles

WEEK 22

Total mileage—35 miles

Mon:	Massage
Tues:	Run 4 miles
Wed:	Run 4 miles
Thurs:	Run 4 miles
Fri:	Weight Training and Yoga
Sat:	Run 20 miles
Sun:	Run 3 miles

WEEK 23

Total mileage—26 miles

Mon:	Massage
Tues:	Run 6 miles
Wed:	Run 5 miles
Thurs:	Run 4 miles
Fri:	Yoga
Sat:	Run 6 miles
Sun:	Run 5 miles

WEEK 24

Total mileage—3 miles+ Race

Mon:	Massage
Tues:	Off
Wed:	Run 3 miles
Thurs:	Off
Friday:	Yoga
Sat:	Off
Sun—Race Day:	26.2 miles

RACE RECOVERY

1. Drink at least 5 cups of water immediately after the race. You can lose up to 10 lbs. of water weight during a race!
2. Keep on your feet for a while—don't sit right away.
3. Eat some fruit, bread, energy bars, or other carbohydrates.
4. Stretch.
5. Put on warm, dry clothes. Shower, if one is available.
6. Massage your muscles.

In the weeks after your marathon, stretch regularly and get massages. Keep your feet elevated when you're resting. Do not resume running or training hard for several weeks.

RACE DAY CHECKLIST

- ☐ Shorts/running tights
- ☐ Shirt (not cotton—take advantage of the new fabrics that wick away sweat yet keep you relatively dry)
- ☐ Socks (see above)
- ☐ Running shoes (avoid the urge to run in a new pair—give your sneakers about 3 weeks of roadwork before the marathon)
- ☐ Visor/cap/sunglasses
- ☐ Race number
- ☐ Safety pins
- ☐ Sunscreen
- ☐ A roll of toilet paper
- ☐ Water bottle
- ☐ Vaseline or Body Glide (for your inner thighs and armpits—any body parts that rub together should be lubricated)
- ☐ Sweat suit to wear after race
- ☐ High-carbohydrate food for after the race
- ☐ Bandages (men should put Band-Aids over their nipples, as this area can become very sensitive and bleed!)
- ☐ Keys
- ☐ Small amount of cash, in case you have to leave race and need money for phone call or cab fare
- ☐ Hair clips
- ☐ Towel
- ☐ Tampons if you're likely to get your period
- ☐ Large plastic garbage bag with hole cut out for your head in case it rains

Good luck . . . train hard . . . and have fun!

APPENDIX A
MARATHON CALENDAR

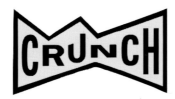

Here's list of marathons in the United States by month. Some marathons have very high entry requirements, so check with the marathon organizers before you show up. You can find more information about the marathons through local chambers of commerce or on the Web. The New York Road Runner's Web site, **www.nyrrc.org**, which provides a list of marathons worldwide, also has links to popular marathons' Web sites.

JANUARY

San Diego Marathon	San Diego, CA
Houston Marathon	Houston, TX

FEBRUARY

Carolina Marathon and 10K	Columbia, SC
Las Vegas Marathon, Half-Marathon, and 5K	Las Vegas, NV
Motorola Austin Marathon	Austin, TX
Cowtown Marathon/10K/5K	Fort Worth, TX

MARCH

City of Los Angeles Marathon/5K	Los Angeles, CA

APRIL

The Army Marathon	Fort Huachuca, AZ
Fred's Marathon and Half-Marathon	Devens, MA
Boston Marathon	Boston, MA
Big Sur Marathon	Carmel, CA

MAY

Pittsburgh Marathon and 10K	Pittsburgh, PA
Rock 'n' Roll Marathon	San Diego, CA
Vermont City Marathon/Relay	Burlington, VT

JUNE

God's Country Adelphia Marathon	Potter County, PA
Hoosier Marathon	Fort Wayne, IN
Grandma's Marathon/ Garry Bjorklund Half	Duluth, MN
Anchorage Marathon	Anchorage, AK
Deseret Marathon and 10K	Salt Lake City, UT

SEPTEMBER

USAF Marathon	Dayton, OH
Fox Cities Marathon	Neenah, WI

OCTOBER

St. George Marathon	St. George, UT
Portland Marathon	Portland, OR
Twin Cities Marathon	Minneapolis/St. Paul, MN
Hartford Marathon	Hartford, CT
Lake Tahoe Marathon	Lake Tahoe, NV
Indianapolis Marathon and Half-Marathon	Indianapolis, IN
Atlantic City Marathon	Atlantic City, NJ
Bay State Marathon and Relay	Lowell, MA
LaSalle Banks Chicago Marathon/5K	Chicago, IL
Marine Corps Marathon	Washington, DC
Cape Cod Marathon	Falmouth, MA

NOVEMBER

New York City Marathon	New York, NY
Crestar Richmond Marathon and Coca-Cola 5 Miler	Richmond, VA
Columbus Marathon	Columbus, OH
Philadelphia Marathon & 8K	Philadelphia, PA

DECEMBER

Honolulu Marathon	Honolulu, HI

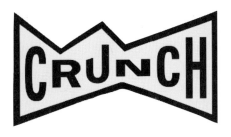

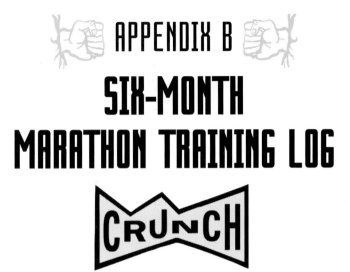

APPENDIX B
SIX-MONTH
MARATHON TRAINING LOG

As we mentioned in Chapter 1, a training log is an invaluable tool. Recording your progress in a place that you can refer back to will contribute to your sense of accomplishment. The log will become a source of motivation—challenging you to stick to your schedule and to figure out ways to overcome shortcomings in your training.

The following log sheets correspond to the weekly training regimen prescribed in this book. Each week, for 24 weeks, fill out the corresponding log sheet. Under "Comments," note the location of your run, the time of day, the time of the run, the weather conditions, and how you felt during and after the run. You can also note what you ate and how much water you drank—and whether you need to change your eating habits for the next run. Next to the strength training exercises, note whether you completed the sets. Next to the cross training days, note the type of cross training you did, and so forth.

Every month, look back over your log. Remind yourself about the obstacles you encountered—be they bad weather conditions, insufficient energy, or pulled muscles—and what you can do to overcome them in the future. And, just as important, remind yourself of the progress you've made.

WEEK 1

DAY	ACTIVITY	COMMENTS
Mon:	Off	
Tues:	Run 1 mile	
Wed:	Weights	

- ❑ Reverse lunges .... 2 x 20 (each leg)
- ❑ Step-ups .... 2 x 20 (each leg)
- ❑ Leg presses .... 2 x 10 (1/2 your weight)
- ❑ Hamstring curls .... 2 x 15
- ❑ Push-ups .... 1 set until exhaustion
- ❑ Pec decks .... 2 x 20
- ❑ Weight-assisted pull-ups .... 1 set until exhaustion
- ❑ Seated rows .... 2 x 20
- ❑ Shoulder presses .... 2 x 20
- ❑ Lateral raises .... 2 x 15
- ❑ Crunches .... 200 (sets of 25 to 50 reps)

Thurs:	Run 1 mile	
Fri:	Yoga	
Sat or Sun:	Long run—3 miles	

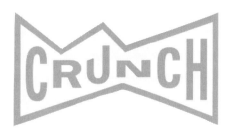

WEEK 2

DAY	ACTIVITY	COMMENTS
Mon:	Off	
Tues:	Run 1 mile	

Wed: **Weights**

- ❑ Reverse lunges .... 2 x 20 (each leg)
- ❑ Step-ups .... 2 x 20 (each leg)
- ❑ Leg presses .... 2 x 10 (1/2 your weight)
- ❑ Hamstring curls .... 2 x 15
- ❑ Push-ups .... 1 set until exhaustion
- ❑ Pec decks .... 2 x 20
- ❑ Weight-assisted pull-ups .... 1 set until exhaustion
- ❑ Seated rows .... 2 x 20
- ❑ Shoulder presses .... 2 x 20
- ❑ Lateral raises .... 2 x 15
- ❑ Crunches .... 200 (sets of 25 to 50)

Thurs:	Run 1 mile	
Fri:	Yoga	
Sat or Sun:	Long run—3 miles	

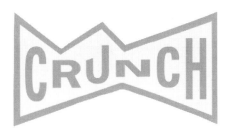

WEEK 3

DAY	ACTIVITY	COMMENTS
Mon:	Off	
Tues:	Run 1 mile	
Wed:	Weights	

- ❑ Reverse lunges .... 2 x 20 (each leg)
- ❑ Step-ups .... 2 x 20 (each leg)
- ❑ Leg presses .... 2 x 10 (1/2 your weight)
- ❑ Hamstring curls .... 2 x 15
- ❑ Push-ups .... 1 set until exhaustion
- ❑ Pec decks .... 2 x 20
- ❑ Weight-assisted pull-ups .... 1 set until exhaustion
- ❑ Seated rows .... 2 x 20
- ❑ Shoulder presses .... 2 x 20
- ❑ Lateral raises .... 2 x 15
- ❑ Crunches .... 200 (sets of 25 to 50)

Thurs:	Run 2 miles	
Fri:	Yoga	
Sat or Sun:	Long run—3 miles	

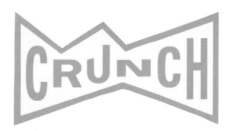

WEEK 4

DAY	ACTIVITY	COMMENTS
Mon:	Off	
Tues:	Run 2 miles	
Wed:	Weights	

- ❏ Reverse lunges .... 2 x 20 (each leg)
- ❏ Step-ups .... 2 x 20 (each leg)
- ❏ Leg presses .... 2 x 10 (1/2 your weight)
- ❏ Hamstring curls .... 2 x 15
- ❏ Push-ups .... 1 set until exhaustion
- ❏ Pec decks .... 2 x 20
- ❏ Weight-assisted pull-ups .... 1 set until exhaustion
- ❏ Seated rows .... 2 x 20
- ❏ Shoulder presses .... 2 x 20
- ❏ Lateral raises .... 2 x 15
- ❏ Crunches .... 200 (sets of 25 to 50)

Thurs:	Run 2 miles	
Fri:	Yoga	
Sat or Sun:	Long run—4 miles	

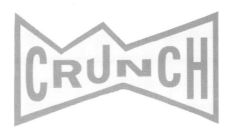

WEEK 5

DAY	ACTIVITY	COMMENTS
Mon:	Off	
Tues:	Run 2 miles	

Wed: Weights

- ❑ Reverse lunges .... 2 x 30 (alternating legs)
- ❑ Step-ups .... 2 x 30 (alternating legs)
- ❑ Leg presses .... 3 x 12 (1/2 your weight)
- ❑ Hamstring curls .... 3 x 15
- ❑ Shoulder presses .... 3 x 20
- ❑ Lateral raises .... 3 x 15
- ❑ Crunches 200

Thurs:	Run 2 miles	
Fri:	Yoga	

Sat: Weights

- ❑ Calf raises .... 2 x 20
- ❑ Hip abductors .... 2 x 20
- ❑ Hip adductors .... 2 x 20
- ❑ Push-ups .... 2 sets until exhaustion
- ❑ Dumbbell bench presses .... 2 x 20
- ❑ Pec decks .... 2 x 20
- ❑ Weight-assisted pull-ups .... 2 sets until exhaustion
- ❑ Seated rows .... 2 x 20
- ❑ Crunches 200

Sun:	Long run—4 miles	

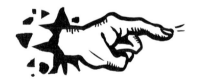

WEEK 6

DAY	ACTIVITY	COMMENTS
Mon:	Off	
Tues:	Run 2 miles	
Wed:	Weights	

- ❏ Reverse lunges .... 2 x 30 (alternating legs)
- ❏ Step-ups .... 2 x 30 (alternating legs)
- ❏ Leg presses .... 3 x 12 (1/2 your weight)
- ❏ Hamstring curls .... 3 x 15
- ❏ Shoulder presses .... 3 x 20
- ❏ Lateral raises .... 3 x 15
- ❏ Crunches 200

Thurs:	Run 3 miles	
Fri:	Yoga	
Sat:	Weights	

- ❏ Calf raises .... 2 x 20
- ❏ Hip abductors .... 2 x 20
- ❏ Hip adductors .... 2 x 20
- ❏ Push-ups .... 2 sets until exhaustion
- ❏ Dumbbell bench presses .... 2 x 20
- ❏ Pec decks .... 2 x 20
- ❏ Weight-assisted pull-ups .... 2 sets until exhaustion
- ❏ Seated rows .... 2 x 20
- ❏ Crunches 200

Sun:	Long run—4 miles	

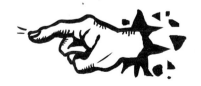

WEEK 7

DAY	ACTIVITY	COMMENTS
Mon:	Off	
Tues:	Run 3 miles	

Wed: Weights

- ❑ Reverse lunges .... 2 x 30 (alternating legs)
- ❑ Step-ups .... 2 x 30 (alternating legs)
- ❑ Leg presses .... 3 x 12 (1/2 your weight)
- ❑ Hamstring curls .... 3 x 15
- ❑ Shoulder presses .... 3 x 20
- ❑ Lateral raises .... 3 x 15
- ❑ Crunches 200

Thurs:	Run 3 mile	
Fri:	Yoga	

Sat: Weights

- ❑ Calf raises .... 2 x 20
- ❑ Hip abductors .... 2 x 20
- ❑ Hip adductors .... 2 x 20
- ❑ Push-ups .... 2 sets until exhaustion
- ❑ Dumbbell bench presses .... 2 x 20
- ❑ Pec decks .... 2 x 20
- ❑ Weight-assisted pull-ups .... 2 sets until exhaustion
- ❑ Seated rows .... 2 x 20
- ❑ Crunches 200

Sun:	Long run—4 miles	

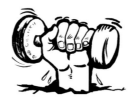

WEEK 8

DAY	ACTIVITY	COMMENTS
Mon:	Off	
Tues:	Run 3 miles	

Wed: Weights

- ❏ Reverse lunges............................. 2 x 30 (alternating legs)
- ❏ Step-ups.. 2 x 30 (alternating legs)
- ❏ Leg presses .... 3 x 12 (1/2 your weight)
- ❏ Hamstring curls........................... 3 x 15
- ❏ Shoulder presses .... 3 x 20
- ❏ Lateral raises .... 3 x 15
- ❏ Crunches 200

Thurs:	Run 3 miles	
Fri:	Yoga	

Sat: Weights

- ❏ Calf raises .... 2 x 20
- ❏ Hip abductors .... 2 x 20
- ❏ Hip adductors .... 2 x 20
- ❏ Push-ups...................................... 2 sets until exhaustion
- ❏ Dumbbell bench presses........... 2 x 20
- ❏ Pec decks.................................... 2 x 20
- ❏ Weight-assisted pull-ups .... 2 sets until exhaustion
- ❏ Seated rows .... 2 x 20
- ❏ Crunches 200

Sun:	Long run—5 miles	

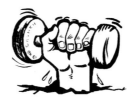

WEEK 9

DAY	ACTIVITY	COMMENTS
Mon:	Off	
Tues:	Interval Training	

- ❑ Walking lunges .... 3 minutes
- ❑ Leg presses .... 1 x 15 (1/2 your weight)
- ❑ Leg presses .... 2 x 8 (your full body weight)
- ❑ Jumping jacks .... 1 minute
- ❑ Leg extensions .... 2 x 15
- ❑ Vertical (or lateral) hops .... 1 minute
- ❑ Push-ups .... 1 set until exhaustion
- ❑ Incline bench presses .... 2 x 12
- ❑ Push-ups .... 1 set until exhaustion
- ❑ Bicep curls .... 2 x 15
- ❑ Crunches 300

Wed:	Run 3 miles	
Thurs:	Cross Training	
Fri:	Interval Training	

- ❑ Weight-assisted pull-ups .... 1 set until exhaustion (1/2 weight)
- ❑ Squat thrusts .... 1 minutes
- ❑ Weight-assisted pull-ups .... 1 set until exhaustion (1/2 weight)
- ❑ Step-ups .... 2 minutes
- ❑ Seated rows .... 2 x 15
- ❑ Hamstring curls .... 1 x 15
- ❑ Plie squats .... 1 x 25 (10 to 25 lbs.)
- ❑ Hamstring curls .... 1 x 15
- ❑ Plie squats .... 1 x 25 (10 to 25 lbs.)
- ❑ Shoulder presses .... 2 x 15
- ❑ Lateral raises .... 2 x 15
- ❑ Calf raises .... 2 x 15
- ❑ Crunches 300

| **Sat:** | Yoga | |
| **Sun:** | Run 5 miles | |

WEEK 10

DAY	ACTIVITY	COMMENTS
Mon:	Off	

Tues: Interval Training

- ❑ Walking lunges .... 3 minutes
- ❑ Leg presses .... 1 x 15 (1/2 your weight)
- ❑ Leg presses .... 2 x 8 (your full body weight)
- ❑ Jumping jacks .... 1 minute
- ❑ Leg extensions .... 2 x 15
- ❑ Vertical (or lateral) hops .... 1 minute
- ❑ Push-ups .... 1 set until exhaustion
- ❑ Incline bench presses .... 2 x 12
- ❑ Push-ups .... 1 set until exhaustion
- ❑ Bicep curls .... 2 x 15
- ❑ Crunches 300

Wed: Run 4 miles

Thurs: Cross Training

Fri: Interval Training

- ❑ Weight-assisted pull-ups .... 1 set until exhaustion (1/2 weight)
- ❑ Squat thrusts .... 1 minutes
- ❑ Weight-assisted pull-ups .... 1 set until exhaustion (1/2 weight)
- ❑ Step-ups .... 2 minutes
- ❑ Seated rows .... 2 x 15
- ❑ Hamstring curls .... 1 x 15
- ❑ Plie squats .... 1 x 25 (10 to 25 lbs.)
- ❑ Hamstring curls .... 1 x 15
- ❑ Plie squats .... 1 x 25 (10 to 25 lbs.)
- ❑ Shoulder presses .... 2 x 15
- ❑ Lateral raises .... 2 x 15
- ❑ Calf raises .... 2 x 15
- ❑ Crunches 300

Sat: Yoga

Sun: Run 5 miles

WEEK 11

DAY	ACTIVITY	COMMENTS
Mon:	Off	
Tues:	Interval Training	

- ❑ Walking lunges .... 3 minutes
- ❑ Leg presses .... 1 x 15 (1/2 your weight)
- ❑ Leg presses .... 2 x 8 (your full body weight)
- ❑ Jumping jacks .... 1 minute
- ❑ Leg extensions .... 2 x 15
- ❑ Vertical (or lateral) hops .... 1 minute
- ❑ Push-ups....................................... 1 set until exhaustion
- ❑ Incline bench presses .... 2 x 12
- ❑ Push-ups....................................... 1 set until exhaustion
- ❑ Bicep curls .... 2 x 15
- ❑ Crunches 300

Wed:	Run 5 miles	
Thurs:	Cross Training	
Fri:	Interval Training	

- ❑ Weight-assisted pull-ups .... 1 set until exhaustion (1/2 weight)
- ❑ Squat thrusts .... 1 minutes
- ❑ Weight-assisted pull-ups .... 1 set until exhaustion (1/2 weight)
- ❑ Step-ups....................................... 2 minutes
- ❑ Seated rows .... 2 x 15
- ❑ Hamstring curls .... 1 x 15
- ❑ Plie squats .... 1 x 25 (using a 10 to 25 lbs.)
- ❑ Hamstring curls .... 1 x 15
- ❑ Plie squats .... 1 x 25 (using a 10 to 25 lbs.)
- ❑ Shoulder presses .... 2 x 15
- ❑ Lateral raises .... 2 x 15
- ❑ Calf raises .... 2 x 15
- ❑ Crunches 300

Sat:	Yoga	
Sun:	Run 5 miles	

WEEK 12

DAY	ACTIVITY	COMMENTS
Mon:	Off	

Tues: Interval Training

- ❏ Walking lunges .... 3 minutes
- ❏ Leg presses .... 1 x 15 (1/2 your weight)
- ❏ Leg presses .... 2 x 8 (your full body weight)
- ❏ Jumping jacks .... 1 minute
- ❏ Leg extensions .... 2 x 15
- ❏ Vertical (or lateral) hops .... 1 minute
- ❏ Push-ups .... 1 set until exhaustion
- ❏ Incline bench presses .... 2 x 12
- ❏ Push-ups .... 1 set until exhaustion
- ❏ Bicep curls .... 2 x 15
- ❏ Crunches 300

Wed: Run 6 miles

Thurs: Cross Training

Fri: Interval Training

- ❏ Weight-assisted pull-ups .... 1 set until exhaustion (1/2 weight)
- ❏ Squat thrusts .... 1 minutes
- ❏ Weight-assisted pull-ups .... 1 set until exhaustion (1/2 weight)
- ❏ Step-ups .... 2 minutes
- ❏ Seated rows .... 2 x 15
- ❏ Hamstring curls .... 1 x 15
- ❏ Plie squats .... 1 x 25 (using a 10 to 25 lbs.)
- ❏ Hamstring curls .... 1 x 15
- ❏ Plie squats .... 1 x 25 (using a 10 to 25 lbs.)
- ❏ Shoulder presses .... 2 x 15
- ❏ Lateral raises .... 2 x 15
- ❏ Calf raises .... 2 x 15
- ❏ Crunches 300

Sat: Yoga

Sun: Run 6 miles

WEEK 13

DAY	ACTIVITY	COMMENTS
Mon:	Off	
Tues:	Interval Training	
Wed:	Run 5 miles	

- ❏ Walking lunges .... 3 minutes
- ❏ Leg presses .... 3 x 12 (your full body weight)
- ❏ Squat thrusts .... 1 minute
- ❏ Weight-assisted pull-ups .... 1 set until exhaustion (1/2 weight)
- ❏ Bicep curls .... 2 x 12
- ❏ Vertical hops .... 1 minute
- ❏ Push-ups .... 1 set until exhaustion
- ❏ Flat bench presses .... 2 x 10
- ❏ Mountain climbers .... 1 minute
- ❏ Hamstring curls .... 2 x 12
- ❏ Plie squats .... 2 x 25   (10 –25 lbs.)
- ❏ Jumping jacks .... 2 minutes
- ❏ Crunches 300

DAY	ACTIVITY	COMMENTS
Thurs:	Off	
Fri:	Cross Training	
Sat:	Yoga	
Sun:	Run 7 miles	

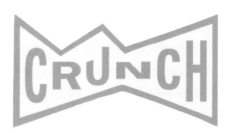

WEEK 14

DAY	ACTIVITY	COMMENTS
Mon:	Off	
Tues:	Interval Training	

- ❏ Walking lunges .... 3 minutes
- ❏ Leg presses .... 3 x 12 (your full body weight)
- ❏ Squat thrusts .... 1 minute
- ❏ Weight-assisted pull-ups .... 1 set until exhaustion (1/2 weight)
- ❏ Bicep curls .... 2 x 12
- ❏ Vertical hops .... 1 minute
- ❏ Push-ups .... 1 set until exhaustion
- ❏ Flat bench presses .... 2 x 10
- ❏ Mountain climbers .... 1 minute
- ❏ Hamstring curls .... 2 x 12
- ❏ Plie squats .... 2 x 25 (10 –25 lbs.)
- ❏ Jumping jacks .... 2 minutes
- ❏ Crunches 300

DAY	ACTIVITY	COMMENTS
Wed:	Run 5 miles	
Thurs:	Off	
Fri:	Cross Training	
Sat:	Yoga	
Sun:	Run 8 miles	

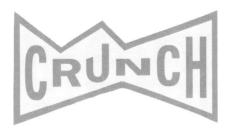

WEEK 15

DAY	ACTIVITY	COMMENTS
Mon:	Off	

Tues: Interval Training
- ❏ Walking lunges .... 3 minutes
- ❏ Leg presses .... 3 x 12 (your full body weight)
- ❏ Squat thrusts .... 1 minute
- ❏ Weight-assisted pull-ups .... 1 set until exhaustion (1/2 weight)
- ❏ Bicep curls .... 2 x 12
- ❏ Vertical hops .... 1 minute
- ❏ Push-ups .... 1 set until exhaustion
- ❏ Flat bench presses .... 2 x 10
- ❏ Mountain climbers .... 1 minute
- ❏ Hamstring curls .... 2 x 12
- ❏ Plie squats .... 2 x 25 (10 –25 lbs.)
- ❏ Jumping jacks .... 2 minutes
- ❏ Crunches 300

Wed:	Run 6 miles	
Thurs:	Off	
Fri:	Cross Training	
Sat:	Yoga	
Sun:	Run 8 miles	

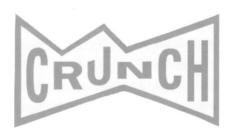

WEEK 16

DAY	ACTIVITY	COMMENTS
Mon:	Off	
Tues:	Interval Training	

- ❑ Walking lunges .... 3 minutes
- ❑ Leg presses .... 3 x 12 (your full body weight)
- ❑ Squat thrusts .... 1 minute
- ❑ Weight-assisted pull-ups .... 1 set until exhaustion (1/2 weight)
- ❑ Bicep curls .... 2 x 12
- ❑ Vertical hops .... 1 minute
- ❑ Push-ups .... 1 set until exhaustion
- ❑ Flat bench presses .... 2 x 10
- ❑ Mountain climbers .... 1 minute
- ❑ Hamstring curls .... 2 x 12
- ❑ Plie squats .... 2 x 25 (10 –25 lbs.)
- ❑ Jumping jacks .... 2 minutes
- ❑ Crunches 300

Wed:	Run 6 miles	
Thurs:	Off	
Fri:	Cross Training	
Sat:	Yoga	
Sun:	Run 9 miles	

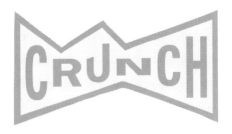

WEEK 17

DAY	ACTIVITY	COMMENTS
Mon:	Massage	
Tues:	Run 4 miles	
Wed:	Run 4 miles	
Thurs:	Run 4 miles	
Fri:	Weight Training and Yoga	

- ❑ Bench presses .... 2 x 20
- ❑ Lat pull-downs .... 2 x 20
- ❑ Leg presses .... 2 x 15
- ❑ Hamstring curls .... 2 x 15
- ❑ Shoulder presses .... 2 x 15
- ❑ Calf raises .... 2 x 15
- ❑ Bicep curls .... 2 x 20
- ❑ Tricep bench dips .... 2 sets to exhaustion

Sat:	Run 10 miles	
Sun:	Run 3 miles	

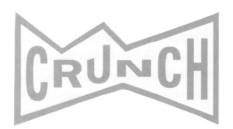

WEEK 18

DAY	ACTIVITY	COMMENTS
Mon:	Off	
Tues:	Run 6 miles	
Wed:	Run 6 miles	
Thurs:	Run 6 miles	

Fri: Weight Training and Yoga

- ❏ Bench presses .... 2 x 20
- ❏ Lat pull-downs .... 2 x 20
- ❏ Leg presses .... 2 x 15
- ❏ Hamstring curls .... 2 x 15
- ❏ Shoulder presses .... 2 x 15
- ❏ Calf raises .... 2 x 15
- ❏ Bicep curls .... 2 x 20
- ❏ Tricep bench dips .... 2 sets to exhaustion

Sat:	Run 14 miles	
Sun:	Run 3 miles	

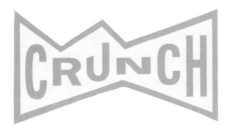

WEEK 19

DAY	ACTIVITY	COMMENTS
Mon:	Massage	
Tues:	Run 6 miles	
Wed:	Run 4 miles	
Thurs:	Run 6 miles	
Fri:	Weight Training and Yoga	

- ❏ Bench presses .... 2 x 20
- ❏ Lat pull-downs .... 2 x 20
- ❏ Leg presses .... 2 x 15
- ❏ Hamstring curls .... 2 x 15
- ❏ Shoulder presses .... 2 x 15
- ❏ Calf raises .... 2 x 15
- ❏ Bicep curls .... 2 x 20
- ❏ Tricep bench dips .... 2 sets to exhaustion

DAY	ACTIVITY	COMMENTS
Sat:	Run 16 miles	
Sun:	Run 4 miles	

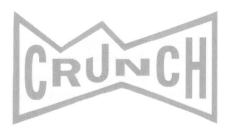

WEEK 20

DAY	ACTIVITY	COMMENTS
Mon:	Off	
Tues:	Run 4 miles	
Wed:	Run 4 miles	
Thurs:	Run 4 miles	

Fri: Weight Training and Yoga

- ❏ Bench presses .... 2 x 20
- ❏ Lat pull-downs .... 2 x 20
- ❏ Leg presses .... 2 x 15
- ❏ Hamstring curls .... 2 x 15
- ❏ Shoulder presses .... 2 x 15
- ❏ Calf raises .... 2 x 15
- ❏ Bicep curls .... 2 x 20
- ❏ Tricep bench dips .... 2 sets to exhaustion

Sat:	Run 20 miles	
Sun:	Off	

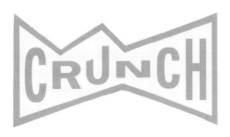

WEEK 21

DAY	ACTIVITY	COMMENTS
Mon:	Massage	
Tues:	Run 4 miles	
Wed:	Run 6 miles	
Thurs:	Run 4 miles	
Fri:	Weight Training and Yoga	

- ❏ Bench presses .... 2 x 20
- ❏ Lat pull-downs .... 2 x 20
- ❏ Leg presses .... 2 x 15
- ❏ Hamstring curls .... 2 x 15
- ❏ Shoulder presses .... 2 x 15
- ❏ Calf raises .... 2 x 15
- ❏ Bicep curls .... 2 x 20
- ❏ Tricep bench dips .... 2 sets to exhaustion

DAY	ACTIVITY	COMMENTS
Sat:	Run 16 miles	
Sun:	Run 3 miles	

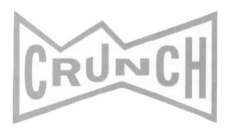

WEEK 22

DAY	ACTIVITY	COMMENTS
Mon:	Massage	
Tues:	Run 4 miles	
Wed:	Run 4 miles	
Thurs:	Run 4 miles	
Fri:	Weight Training and Yoga	

- ❑ Bench presses .... 2 x 20
- ❑ Lat pull-downs .... 2 x 20
- ❑ Leg presses .... 2 x 15
- ❑ Hamstring curls .... 2 x 15
- ❑ Shoulder presses .... 2 x 15
- ❑ Calf raises .... 2 x 15
- ❑ Bicep curls .... 2 x 20
- ❑ Tricep bench dips .... 2 sets to exhaustion

DAY	ACTIVITY	COMMENTS
Sat:	Run 20 miles	
Sun:	Run 3 miles	

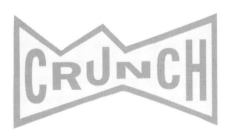

WEEK 23

DAY	ACTIVITY	COMMENTS
Mon:	Massage	
Tues:	Run 6 miles	
Wed:	Run 5 miles	
Thurs:	Run 4 miles	
Fri:	Yoga	
Sat:	Run 6 miles	
Sun:	Run 5 miles	

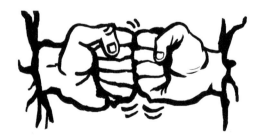

WEEK 24

DAY	ACTIVITY	COMMENTS
Mon:	Massage	
Tues:	Off	
Wed:	Run 3 miles	
Thurs:	Off	
Friday:	Yoga	
Sat:	Off	
Sun	RACE DAY: 26.2 MILES	

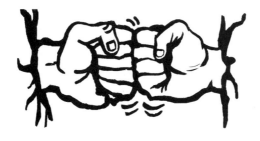

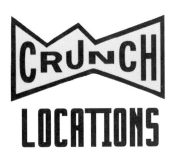

LOCATIONS

Where to work out, pretend to work out, or just stand around calling our personal trainers "Hans" and "Franz" under your breath.

NEW YORK CITY

404 Lafayette Street
(Astor Place and 4th Avenue)
212.614.0120

54 East 13th Street
(University and Broadway)
212.475.2018

162 West 83rd Street
(Columbus and Amsterdam)
212.875.1902

623 Broadway (at Houston)
212.420.0507

152 Christopher Street
(at Greenwich Street)
212.366.3725

1109 Second Avenue
(at 59th Street)
212.758.3434

144 W. 38th St.
(7th Ave. & Broadway)
212.869.7788

LOS ANGELES

8000 Sunset Blvd.
(West Hollywood)
323.654.4550

SAN FRANCISCO

1000 Van Ness Avenue
(Geary and O'Farrell)
415.931.1100

MISSION VIEJO

The Kaleidoscope Center
27741 Crown Valley Parkway
949.582.8181

MIAMI

1259 Washington Avenue
(South Beach)
305.674.8222

ATLANTA AREA
[ALL LOCATIONS: 800.660.5433]

Crunch Club Cobb
North by NW Office Park
1775 Water Place
Atlanta, GA 30339

Crunch Gwinnett
Gwinnett Prado
2300 Pleasant Hill Road
Duluth, GA 30136

Crunch Town Center
Main Street Shopping Center
2600 Prado Lane
Marietta, GA 30066

Crunch Roswell
Roswell Exchange
11060 Alpharetta Highway
Roswell, GA 30076

Crunch Buckhead
3365 Piedmont Road, Suite 1010
Atlanta, GA

Crunch Stone Mountain
Stone Mountain Square
5370 Highway 78 South
Stone Mountain, GA 30087

CHICAGO

Crunch Chicago
350 North State Street
Chicago, IL 60610
312.527.8100

TOKYO

Crunch Omotesando
4-3-24 Jingumae Sibuya

Coming soon to Las Vegas!

Visit us on the Web at
www.crunch.com

Have questions about this workout?

Ask the authors at:

WWW.GETFITNOW.COM

*The **hottest** fitness spot on the internet!*

FEATURING ...

"Ask the Expert" Q&A Boards
Stimulating Discussion groups
Cool Links
Great Photos
Full-Motion Videos
Downloads
The Five Star Fitness Team
Hot Product Reviews
And More!

**Log on today to receive a FREE catalog
or call us at
1-800-906-1234**

Personal Training Coupon

15% OFF! 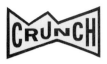 15% OFF!

IT'S EASY . . . Come into any CRUNCH location and receive 15% off your first purchase of personal training. Then just sign, date, and present this coupon at the fitness desk to set up your session.

_____   _____
MEMBER NAME   SIGNATURE

_____   _____
TRAINER NAME   TRAINER SIGNATURE

_____
DATE OF SESSION

Cannot be combined with any other offer. Valid for one use only

- - - - - - - - - - CUT AT DOTTED LINE - - - - - - - - - -

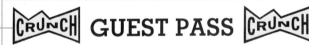 GUEST PASS

$22 value!

Must show picture ID to use facility.
The same guest may use only two guest passes per year

_____   _____
MEMBERSHIP REP   EXPIRATION DATE

OUR MISSION AND PHILOSOPHY

We at CRUNCH warmly welcome people from all walks of life,
regardless of shape, size, sex, or ability.
People don't have to be flawless to feel at home at CRUNCH. We don't care
if our members are 18 or 80, fat or thin, short or tall, muscular or mushy, blond or bald,
or anywhere in between. CRUNCH is not competitive, it is non-judgmental,
it is not elitist, it does not represent a kind of person.
CRUNCH is a gym; a movement which is growing as we continue to perfect our ability
to create an environment where our members don't feel self-conscious,
and don't worry about what others think.
At the heart of CRUNCH's core stands a tremendously experienced and energetic staff
dedicated to creating an environment where everyone feels accepted—
a truly unique place!

WWW.CRUNCH.COM

The **hottest** fitness spot on the internet!

OUR MISSION AND PHILOSOPHY

We at CRUNCH warmly welcome people from all walks of life,
regardless of shape, size, sex, or ability.
People don't have to be flawless to feel at home at CRUNCH. We don't care
if our members are 18 or 80, fat or thin, short or tall, muscular or mushy, blond or bald,
or anywhere in between. CRUNCH is not competitive, it is non-judgmental,
it is not elitist, it does not represent a kind of person.
CRUNCH is a gym; a movement which is growing as we continue to perfect our ability
to create an environment where our members don't feel self-conscious,
and don't worry about what others think.
At the heart of CRUNCH's core stands a tremendously experienced and energetic staff
dedicated to creating an environment where everyone feels accepted—
a truly unique place!

WWW.CRUNCH.COM

The **hottest** fitness spot on the internet!

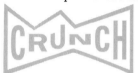

- - - - - - - - - - - CUT AT DOTTED LINE - - - - - - - - - - -

NEW YORK CITY

404 Lafayette Street
(Astor Place and 4th Street)
212.614.0120

54 East 13th Street
(University and Broadway)
212.475.2018

162 West 83rd Street
(Columbus and Amsterdam)
212.875.1902

623 Broadway (at Houston)
212.420.0507

152 Christopher Street
(at Greenwich Street)
212.366.3725

1109 Second Avenue
(at 59th Street)
212.758.3434

144 W. 38th St.
(7th Ave. & Broadway)
212.869.7788

LOS ANGELES

8000 Sunset Blvd.
(West Hollywood)
323.654.4550

SAN FRANCISCO

1000 Van Ness Avenue
(Geary and O'Farrell)
415.931.1100

MISSION VIEJO

The Kaleidoscope Center
27741 Crown Valley
  Parkway
949.582.8181

MIAMI

1259 Washington Avenue
(South Beach)
305.674.8222

ATLANTA AREA
(All locations: 800.660.5433)

Crunch Club Cobb
North by NW Office Park
1775 Water Place
Atlanta, GA 30339

Crunch Gwinnett
Gwinnett Prado
2300 Pleasant Hill Road
Duluth, GA 30136

Crunch Town Center
Main Street Shopping
  Center
2600 Prado Lane
Marietta, GA 30066

Crunch Roswell
Roswell Exchange
11060 Alpharetta Highway
Roswell, GA 30076

Crunch Buckhead
3365 Piedmont Road,
Suite 1010
Atlanta, GA

Crunch Stone Mountain
Stone Mountain Square
5370 Highway 78 South
Stone Mountain, GA 30087

CHICAGO

Crunch Chicago
350 North State Street
Chicago, IL 60610
312.527.8100

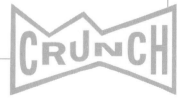

LAS VEGAS COMING SOON!